W0082179

kama sutra52

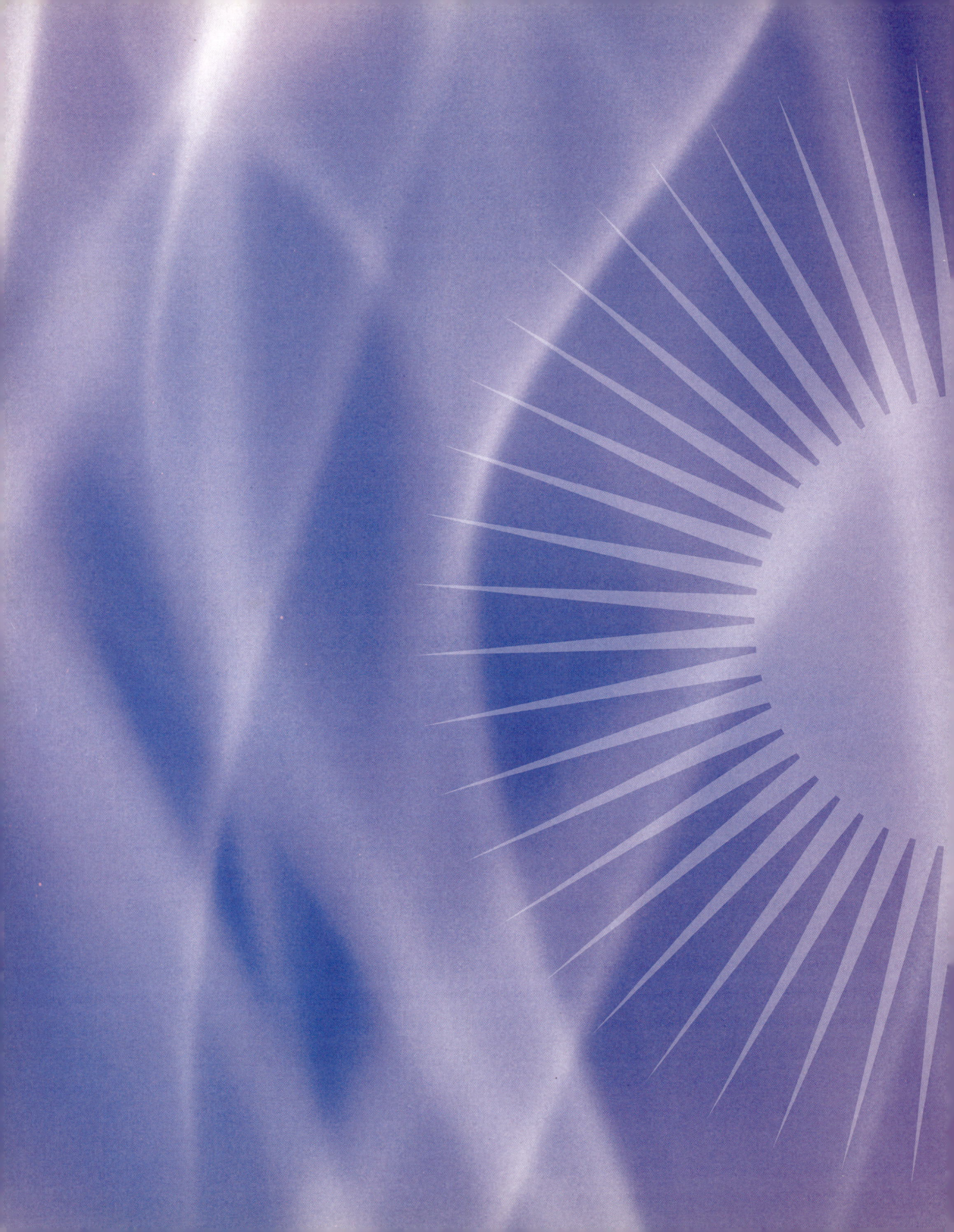

kama sutra52

A YEAR'S WORTH OF THE BEST POSITIONS FOR PASSION AND PLEASURE

Lisa Schrader

Sacred Sexuality Coach
Seen on *The Oprah Winfrey Show*

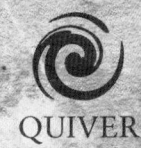

QUIVER

Text © 2009 Lisa Schrader
Photography © 2009 Quiver

First published in the USA in 2009 by
Quiver, a member of
Quayside Publishing Group
100 Cummings Center
Suite 406-L
Beverly, MA 01915-6101
www.quiverbooks.com

All rights reserved. No part of this book may be reproduced or utilized, in any form or by any means, electronic or mechanical, without prior permission in writing from the publisher.

The Publisher maintains the records relating to images in this book required by 18 USC 2257. Records are located at Rockport Publishers, Inc., 100 Cummings Center, Suite 406-L, Beverly, MA 01915-6101.

13 12 11 10 09   1 2 3 4 5

ISBN-13: 978-1-59233-397-4
ISBN-10: 1-59233-397-4

Library of Congress Cataloging-in-Publication Data
Schrader, Lisa.
  Kama sutra 52 : a year's worth of the best positions for passion and pleasure / Lisa Schrader.
     p. cm.
  ISBN-13: 978-1-59233-397-4
  ISBN-10: 1-59233-397-4
  1. Sex instruction. 2. Love. 3. Sexual excitement. 4. Vatsyayana. Kamasutra. I. Title.
  HQ31.S379 2009
  613.9'6—dc22

                                                         2009010351

Cover and book design: Carol Holtz, Holtz Design
Photography: Richard Avery

Printed and bound in Singapore

To the Sacred Marriage of Shiva
and Shakti within each of us
and on the planet as a whole.

contents

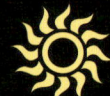

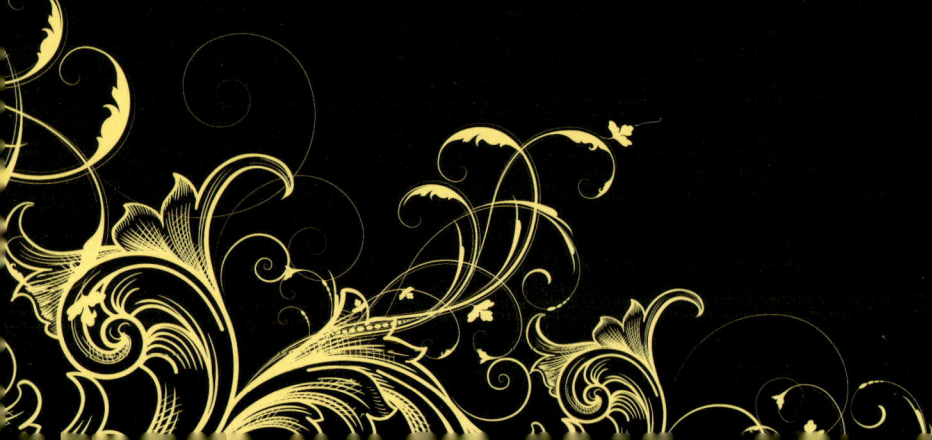

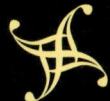

flame

fire

wild fire

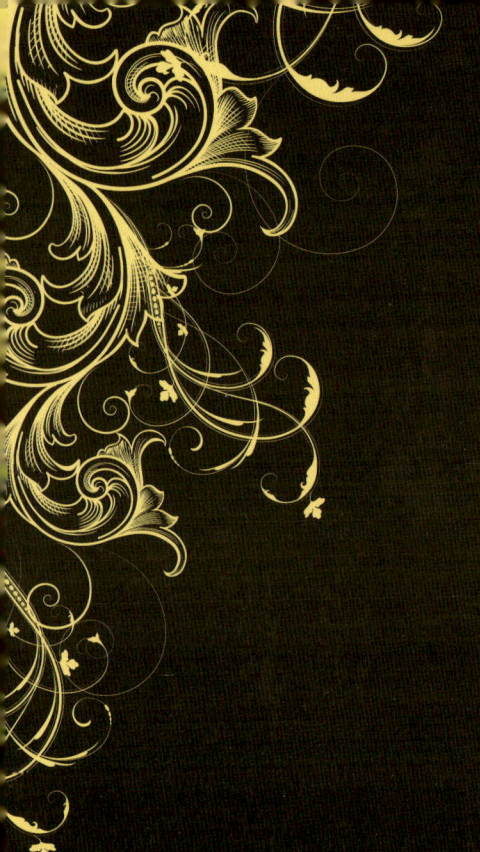

"Out beyond ideas of
wrong-doing and right-
doing there is a field.
I'll meet you there."
—RUMI

The Burning "Yes"

AN OPENING INVITATION

The Kama Sutra, the ancient book of love from India, invites you to come to your senses. Notice the pattern of moonlight on your lover's undulating body. Hear the breath quickening with passion. Inhale the moist scent of desire. Taste the nectar. Feel the melting of skin into skin, all separation dissolving.

Pleasure can awaken you and bring you home. It can release you from the insanity of the mind and usher you back into the wisdom of the body. Alive in your senses, you arrive in the present moment, where all manner of miracles awaits you. Here you turn to your lover and, in a holy moment, discover true communion. Two souls mirroring each other. You feel an eternal essence looking at you through your lover's eyes, and it's the same essence looking through your own eyes. A shiver of recognition moves up your spine and you smile. There you are, breathing into bliss with your beloved when suddenly everything expands, a quantum shift. The bottom falls away, and you find yourself suspended in ecstatic joy. Infinitely simple and clear: the hum and awe of All One.

Is this God?

Is this Love?

Is this Orgasm?

Yes. Yes. Yes.

Maybe it's just the sacred "Yes" of Life.

You name it.

What I do know is that this is the power that changes the world and always has. It lives in you. Pleasure can guide you there. Welcome home.

Blessings on your loving,

Lisa

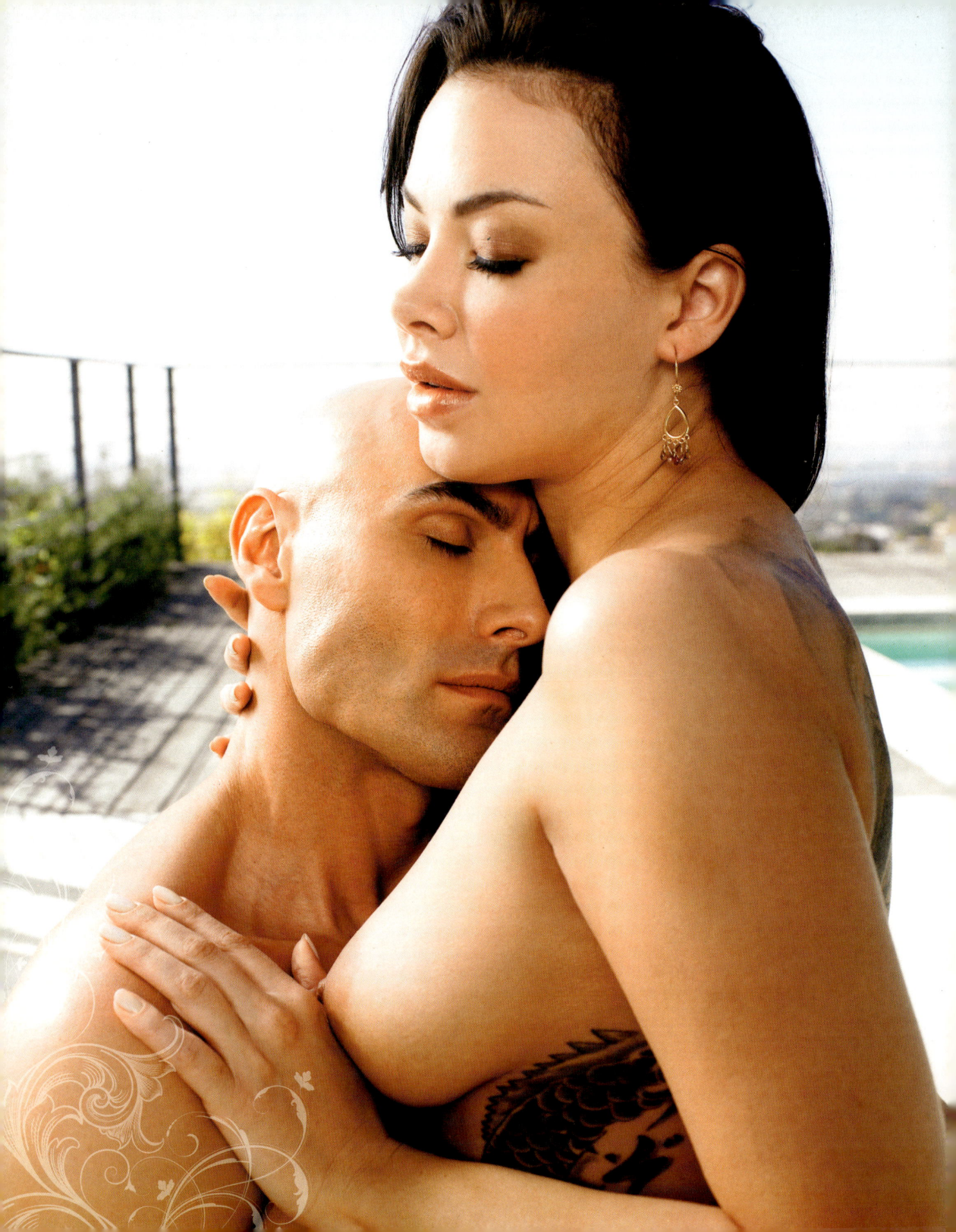

PART I:
Illumination from the Book of Love

AN INTRODUCTION
TO THE KAMA SUTRA

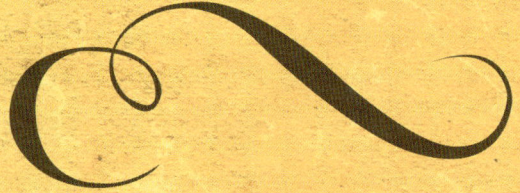

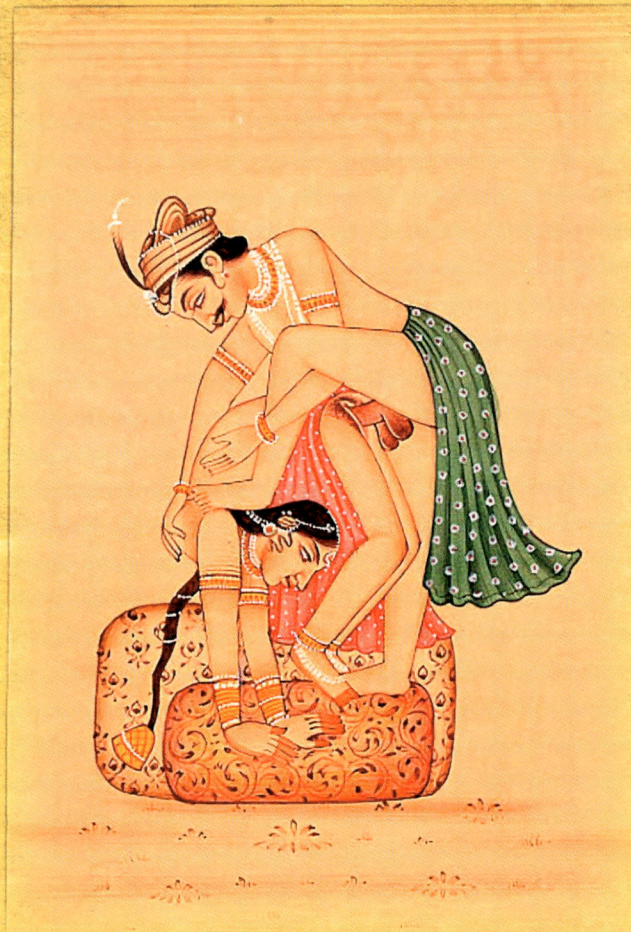

THE KAMA SUTRA REMINDS US of a time when lovemaking was honored as an integral part of the tapestry of life. Sexuality was studied as an art and a science. The exploration of "kama," or pleasure, was one of the cornerstones of being a balanced citizen on the path toward spiritual realization. This certainly has not been our lineage in the West. Perhaps this is one reason why this ancient book of love continues to capture our imagination.

The Kama Sutra can be viewed as an antidote to what ails us. We have become so accustomed to a frenetic pace of life that we feel fortunate if we "squeeze" in sex for a few moments at the end of an exhausting day. We spend money on a dizzying array of entertainment options, but the Kama Sutra takes us back to a time when the hours spent in lovemaking were a primary form of recreation—not only free of charge but good for body, mind, and spirit as well. As much "letting go" as we may have done with our inheritance of sexual guilt and shame, we may still have residual negative ideas about sensual pleasure. Most of us don't automatically think of our sexuality as an integral part of our spiritual development, as one of the most direct routes to God.

THE DESIRE FOR MORE

You're reading this book because you want to explore and learn more about sexuality. It could be that you're happy with your sex life and just want some creative new ideas on how to put two bodies together. If so, you'll find 52 different ways to do that in the positions that follow, complete with detailed descriptions and photos to show you how. That's a year's worth of excitement, fun, and new ideas for erotic play. There's something for everyone, and you don't have to know a thing about the Kama Sutra to thoroughly enjoy yourself.

Others of you want that *plus* a little more. Maybe your sex life has been satisfactory but you hear a whisper (maybe it's a yell) that there's more to it than what you've experienced. You've got the basics down but you know you're hanging out on the tip of the iceberg, that there's an entire world of passion and transformation awaiting you under the surface. Not only do you want to go to the depths (and heights) of your own sexuality, but you want to give that gift to your partner as well. Rock on!

To truly reach a new level of intimacy, magic, and passion, you have to add a few more ingredients. The content in these opening chapters will give you ideas and tools you need to get there, as will the sidebar articles throughout the book.

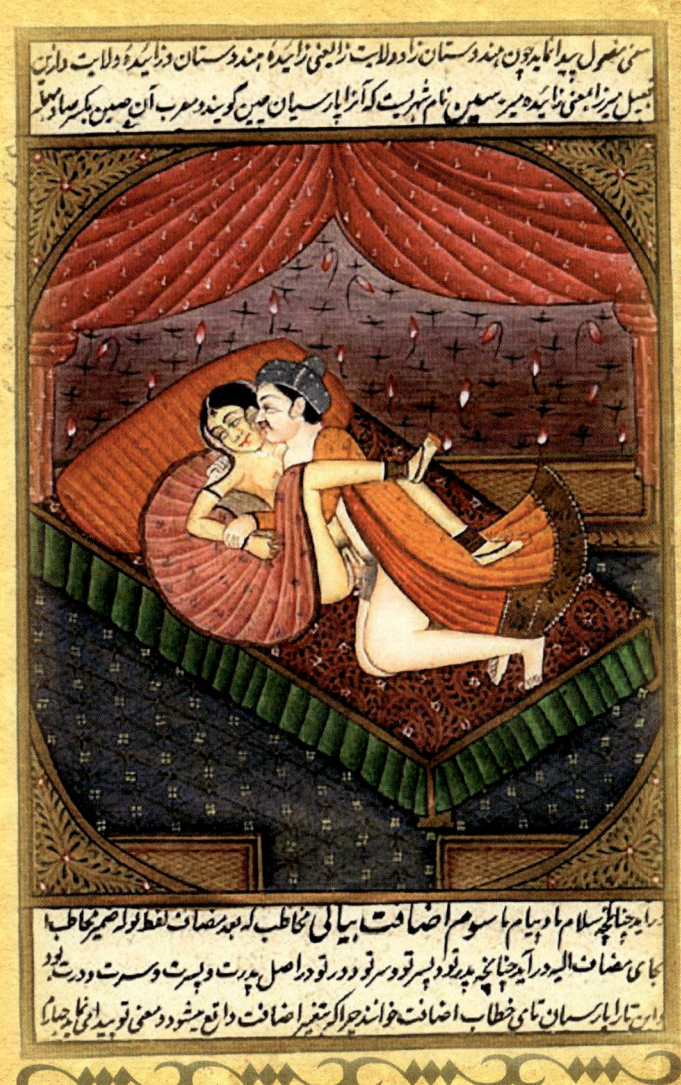

THE TENETS OF THE KAMA SUTRA

The following are some major themes from the Kama Sutra, from the ancient Eastern spiritual philosophy of Tantra, and from sacred sexual practices that I think will most positively impact your own sexual awakening and enjoyment.

SEX IS SACRED

Renowned author Deepak Chopra says, "The truth about sex, and love in general, is that it remains the most powerful spiritual experience that most of us will have in our lifetimes." In fact, "Oh my God" is the most common utterance during orgasm because it is a moment (or hopefully longer) where your identity of "self" disappears and you have the experience of "no-thing-ness," which for a lot of people feels like a return to God. You feel at one with yourself and your partner, without separation. It was most likely such a moment that ushered in your very own conception.

We have all suffered from the tragic divorce between sex and spirit that is our current cultural inheritance. I believe it is our work to heal that division and invite the sacred back into our lovemaking. When we do that, we access the full expression of our eroticism.

How exactly do you do that? You can start by calling in a higher power (whatever that is for you) and ask for blessings on your lovemaking. Then relax, open, and allow yourself to receive it. Ask that your sexuality and orgasmic life force be used by the Divine as a conduit for bringing greater love, energy, and spirit into the physical world. You can do this by yourself, silently. You can also do a short or long ritual with your partner: Create an altar, meditate for a few moments together, and speak your intentions and dedication out loud. In the very potent moment of orgasm, you can tap into the power of sexual magic and supercharge your manifestation abilities by releasing an intention.

The essence of who we are *is* divine, whether we remember it or not. I invite you to simply allow it to shine through you and recognize it in your partner while you make love. Whether you're having a hot, passionate throw-down moment or you're floating for hours on clouds of orgasmic bliss, let your sexuality be a celebration and embodiment of the sacred.

OPEN THE HEART OF SEX

When we open the heart and risk the vulnerability of sharing our tender emotional world with our partner, we engage in "in-to-me-you-see" which takes our sexual "intimacy" to a whole new level. To try this, draw your attention to and breathe deeply into your heart, expand your capacity to give and receive love, and speak what's in your heart to your partner.

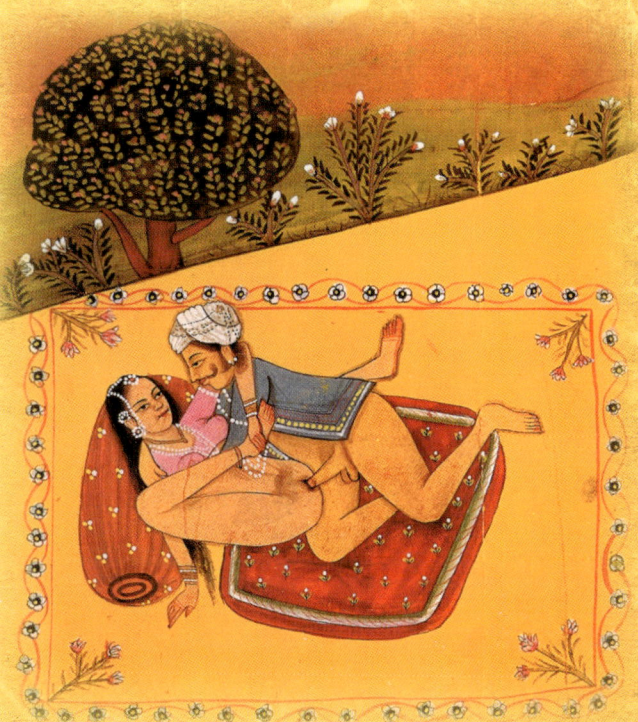

"Unconditional" means loving no matter what the circumstances. It has to start with you loving *you*, and that *includes* loving your body. Regardless of how you feel about your body, it serves you faithfully. And if you think about it, you don't get to enjoy it all that long—barely a blip on the timeline of existence. It's my sincere hope that you fall in love with your body, accepting it exactly the way that it is and *is not*. Don't compare yourself with the models you see in these pages—the oak tree doesn't compare itself with the bamboo—get on with loving what you have and loving the one you're with.

When we really boil it all down, there is only love and fear. There are lots of words we use to describe and dissect our emotions, but the essence is either love or fear. And love can put her arms around the fear, loving it because it is. Invite your heart to guide you on your sexual journey.

PLEASURE IS ENERGY

Not only is sexual pleasure your birthright, but it's good for you, too. The health benefits of being orgasmic and having an active sex life are now well documented by science, psychology, and medicine. Your body was born an expert on ecstasy and sensuality. Just watch a baby for a while and you'll see how his whole world revolves around senses—being held and touched, crying when he needs to be heard, and swallowing sweetness from the breast. Along the

way, culture, religion, and perhaps well-meaning but misguided adults drove us away from our inner body wisdom. Other fear-based ideas of shame, guilt, and separation replaced our sacred relationship with our body's pleasure. The good news is that you can go home again.

No doubt about it, sexual pleasure *can* also lead you astray, feed addictions, and fuel shallow or unconscious impulses (we're human). Sexual pleasure is energy, and just like any kind of energy, it is not inherently good or bad. Electricity, for example, can be used to bring light to the darkness or take a man's life away. There's a good reason that sexuality has been so violently repressed over the ages—it's the most powerful energy that we have access to.

Because of our fear of the potency of sexual pleasure, we tend to either repress it or overindulge as a way to get "control" over it. Both repressing and indulging are actually the same response but in different extremes, two sides of the proverbial coin. The alternative is the "middle way," where we engage with pleasure and enjoy it fully with gratitude and consciousness, without becoming overly attached to it or trying to control it. A tricky balance for sure, and one we deal with in all areas of our life, not just sexuality.

HONOR THE FEMININE

Another key message to be found in the Kama Sutra and other ancient sacred sex philosophies is the emphasis on the inherent equality of masculine and feminine energy. We all possess an inner "sacred marriage" of yin and yang qualities. We are emerging from centuries dominated by the masculine, but now the divine feminine, or "Shakti," is awakening from her slumber to take her rightful place again alongside the masculine. Men and women have both suffered with her absence. It's not just about men honoring women; it's also about women honoring the feminine. In our quest for greater power and equality (a healthy and necessary balancing), many women have lost touch with the inner goddess and the power of her sensual, earthy, intuitive cycles.

Given that he was writing more than two thousand years ago from a very "penis-centric" point of view, it's remarkable how much emphasis Vatsyayana, the author of the Kama Sutra, placed on

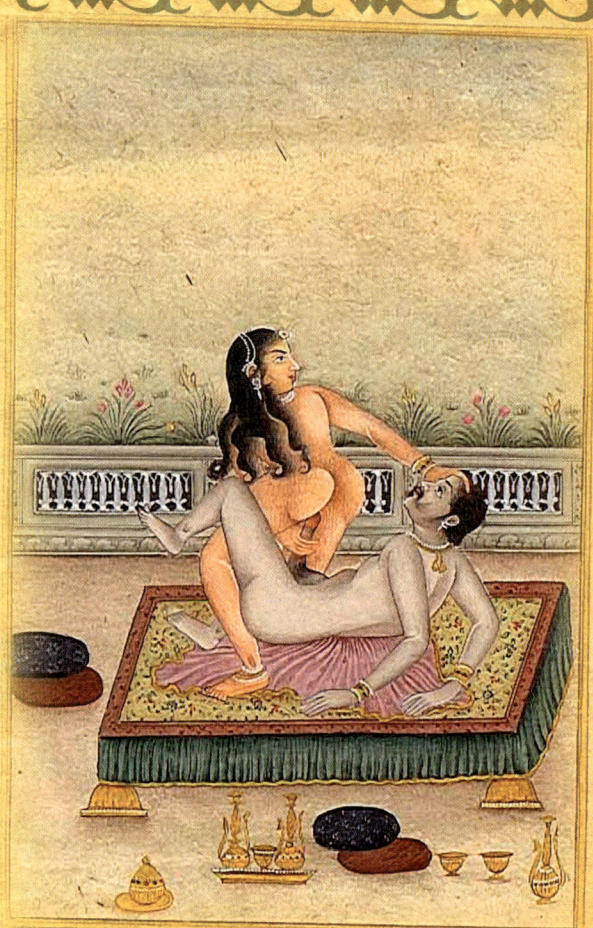

the importance of women's arousal cycles. If you think of the Kama Sutra as a marital guide written for a predominately male audience, this just makes good sense: If it feels good to her, she'll be a more willing participant, and you'll get more sex. Although the sexual content in the original text has a tunnel-vision focus on intercourse solutions, it does address the age-old challenge of the discrepancy between a man's sexual responsiveness (quick to fire) and a woman's temperament (slow to warm). Tantric practices can teach men how to have orgasms without ejaculating and emphasize both partners slowing down to enjoy expanded states of orgasmic pleasure rather than having a goal-oriented race to the big "O" finish line. Having said that, though, doesn't mean that getting it on and getting off quickly can't also be a Tantric experience.

The ancient sacred sexuality writers commonly agreed that a woman's sexual appetite and capacity, once awakened, could surpass that of any man. There is a reason men want so desperately to get inside: They know that therein lies a sacred gateway between heaven and earth. And women need the strong, clear, conscious sacred masculine to help us blossom in that capacity. It takes time, trust, and openness, but the places you will go together as a result of honoring and awakening Shakti will transform you both beyond what you can possibly imagine.

GRACE DESCENDS IN ECSTASY

You can't read about ecstasy and "make" it happen any more than you can read about water and have it quench your thirst. To know water, you have to drink it and swim in it and feel how it is you (given that it's what you're mostly made of). You can read about the positions in this book because doing so is fun and gives you some ideas, but ultimately you have to become fully present with your beloved, stop the insanity of either indulging or fighting the mind, and feel your heart beating and your breath moving in and out. Invite Spirit into your lovemaking and dedicate your union to the betterment of yourself

and the world. That doesn't guarantee ecstasy, but it does go a long way toward preparing the circumstances for its arrival. Ecstasy comes as a form of grace usually when we stop doing and just allow.

RESPECT THE FIRE

Know that your sexual energy doesn't just reside below the waist. It is your life force and enlivens your whole body. Your sexual energy can be used as "rocket fuel" to accelerate any aspect of your life. You can walk around feeling waves of orgasmic energy, love, and gratitude as your way of being (the pro and con is that you will become highly attractive to others). You can use this energy, on an authentic Tantric path, as a fast track to realizing your enlightenment. The point is that it's highly potent, it's yours, and it's up to you how to use it. Be as conscious and intentional as you possibly can. What do you want to fuel in your life right now? What would best serve you, your relationship, and your family?

May your celebration of pleasure open your heart and fuel your highest dreams.

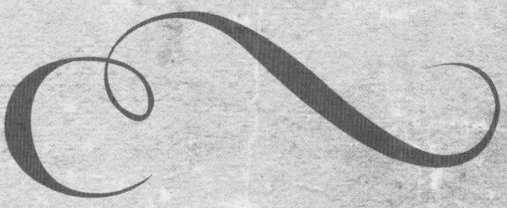

CONTEXT FROM THE ORIGINAL KAMA SUTRA TEXT

It was more than 2,000 years ago that Vatsyayana, a religious monk and scholar, created the original Kama Sutra by reviewing a vast array of ancient writings, religious teachings, and word-of-mouth stories on the many ways of love. Not only did he compile these teachings, but he also added his own colorful commentary, idiosyncratic opinions, and distinctive humor. Perhaps part of the reason that the book has endured as one of the most widely read books ever written on the subject of sexuality and love is that it isn't morality from some dried-up celibate monk. Vatsyayana readily admits that he has followed its "ways of enjoyment." He knows of what he speaks.

PLEASURE IS A WORTHY PURSUIT

I already mentioned that "kama" refers to "pleasure," and a "sutra" is a short lesson. So basically, the original Kama Sutra was a book of teachings on pleasure, also commonly translated as "Aphorisms on Love." Vatsyayana addresses sexuality in detail, given that it is one of life's primary pleasures, although the famous content on sex positions from the original text makes up only a small percentage of the copy and isn't overly descriptive. Modern readers would probably find the original illustrations more erotic and useful than the text.

So why has it continued to capture our attention and inspire us more than 2,000 years later? Perhaps what makes the book so powerful and relevant even today is the philosophy that pleasure from the five senses is integral to our wholeness. Rather than being shameful or needing to be suppressed, sensual pleasure in the Kama Sutra is to be celebrated and explored in a balance with the other guiding principles of success and virtue as a pathway to spiritual liberation.

Although the Kama Sutra honors sexual love and pleasure, it's not a manifesto on hedonism or indulgence. Vatsyayana cautions that "this work is not intended to be used merely as an instrument for satisfying our desires." The focus is on balance: "an intelligent and prudent person," who honors pleasure "without becoming the slave of his passions, obtains success in everything he may undertake."

MEN AND WOMEN DESERVE EQUAL FULFILLMENT

Another remarkable aspect to the Kama Sutra, given that it was written during a time when religious practices prevented women from studying, is Vatsyayana's encouragement of women to learn as much as possible about the practices, because "even the bare knowledge of them gives attractiveness to a woman." Meanwhile, he says that a man acquainted

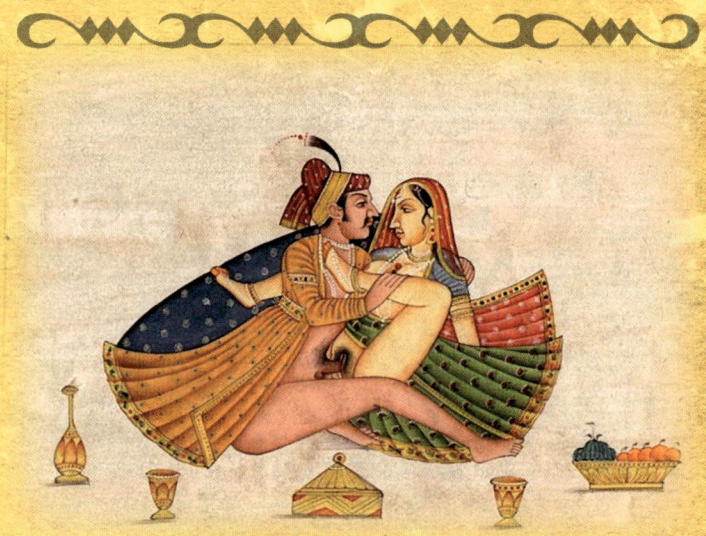

with the practices "gains very soon the hearts of women." In this way, he encourages an equal playing field for men and women, going into detail about women "playing the part of a man" in sexual positions to add variety and as a way to tap into their power and passion during lovemaking. Always there is emphasis on both sexes being entitled to sexual fulfillment and enjoyment.

THE KAMA SUTRA IS A PRODUCT OF ITS TIME

The original text is, however, a product of its time, complete with practices and ideas that are irrelevant or unacceptable today. In the Kama Sutra, it's justifiable to kill a husband and steal his wife, for example, but only if you're so desperately in love with the woman that your own health has deteriorated and you're at risk of dying yourself. Then there's that pesky polygamy and harem problem: The women will have to resort to satisfying themselves "by means of bulbs, roots, and fruits having the form of the lingam (penis)" and will sneak "men into their apartments in the disguise or dress of women" if the king can't deliver.

Mostly, though, the original book of love is full of very practical advice for maintaining harmonious relationships and marriages. Courtship and seduction practices are elaborately detailed, even more so than the intercourse positions. This includes how to decipher what a woman is thinking, when to kiss her and how, the hazards of moving too quickly and making her dislike sex forever, and how fighting, biting, and hitting in a lover's quarrel can generate passion.

NATURE IS REVERED

Because Vatsyayana wrote during a time when people were far more intimate with nature, many of the postures are named after animals, landscapes, and elemental forces. You may find yourself inspired to tap into your own natural rhythm and animal awareness in your lovemaking. You'll find classic Kama Sutra intercourse (or "congress") positions included here, along with many more "Kama Sutra-inspired" positions based on yogic and Tantric sexual practices from the East. I've included content that I think is most relevant to today's lovers looking for new ideas to heat things up in the bedroom and those longing for the deeper fulfillment to be had by entering into the heart and soul of sexual union.

PRACTICAL TIPS FOR GETTING STARTED

This book is organized into four sections: Spark, Flame, Fire, and Wild Fire, with the positions becoming increasingly more challenging. Although some may seem daunting at first, remember that the readers of the original Kama Sutra were likely very adept at yoga. Yoga and spiritual practices were simply a given part of everyday life.

LISTEN TO YOUR BODY

Some of the positions, particularly in the latter sections, require flexibility, strength, and focus. Go slowly, build up your confidence to tackle the more advanced positions when you're ready, and remember that you can have a mind-blowing orgasmic experience with your partner in any position or *without any position at all*. The position itself is just an outer form—it's what happens *inside* with your intention, heart, and energy that makes for the most powerful union. Also be sure to listen to your body and speak honestly with your partner about your capacity and comfort level. Remember, this is the book of *pleasure* we're talking about, so if it hurts, stop.

It's my hope that you'll use the positions to spark your own ideas. Experiment by creating your own or modifying the ones that you like. Although I'm very committed to my own yoga practice, there are positions that don't appeal to me, don't work for my anatomy, or are simply beyond my current ability.

The same will likely be true for you and your partner. In addition to personal preference, bodies come in all shapes and sizes, so some postures may just not "line up" right for you—that doesn't necessarily mean that you're doing it "wrong," just that it's not the best position for you or that it needs some tweaking. Take it all lightly. If you think about it, two people having sex can be pretty ridiculous and funny looking. Perhaps even more so when they're overly serious about getting into some advanced Kama Sutra contortion! Remember to bring your sense of humor to the bedroom.

TRY OUT NEW "DOWN THERE" WORDS

Good communication is a cornerstone of being a great lover. Not only are most of us afraid to let it rip and be vocal during lovemaking, but most of us also find talking about sex embarrassing. Our ability to name a thing and speak about it is the beginning of our power. Reclaim your voice and start talking openly about sex with your partner. When your mental "gremlins" start harassing you with thoughts of embarrassment and shame, simply notice those thoughts and ask yourself whether you can positively know that they are true. You'll be able to identify a gremlin because of the harsh and critical tone of the message. That is not your higher self because it would never speak to you that way. Your true voice celebrates you for being the brilliant child of God that you are—loving every part of you, including your glorious and sensual body.

Our limited vocabulary options also complicate matters. We have a choice between slang words or medical terminology. It's just awkward for most of us to use the words *penis* and *vagina*. Even those of us who are sex educators and very sex-positive can't help but have some baggage attached to those words. They make us snicker. They conjure images of white lab coats, humorless professors, and clinical settings. So rather than trying to "get over" all that's attached to those words, try adopting some new ones.

The Kama Sutra sees the sex organs not just as organs of pleasure; they're also sacred. What a difference from thinking of them as "dirty" or "bad" or "dangerous" in some way. How could our genitalia be anything but sacred? Here is the origin of life. The magnificent flash of light, the oneness of orgasm, which in some totally miraculous way opens the veil between the physical and nonphysical realms, and life *itself* is ushered onto the planet. Then inside the womb, life grows and develops in its own cosmic and floating universe until one day it presses through the magical tunnel into the light and a baby is born.

You bet we need some new words to honor the enormity of that.

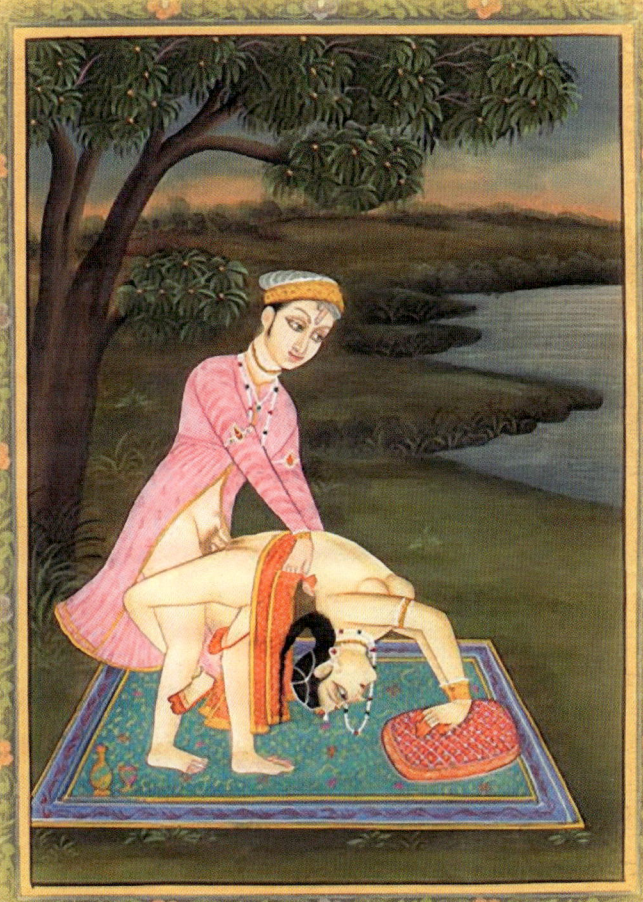

The Sacred Cave

Yoni means "sacred place" or "source." Yoni is considered to be the dwelling place, the sacred temple, of the great goddess Shakti herself. I'm not sure whether you locate your "soul" in any particular place in your body, but I've come to consider my yoni to be the seat of my soul (she sort of radiates out from there). It's *your* job, ladies, to start treating your yoni like a sacred temple. Then you're more likely to attract similar veneration from your partner, or at least be better able to teach him how to pleasure you.

What would you do if you started to think of your yoni as sacred? How would your choices be

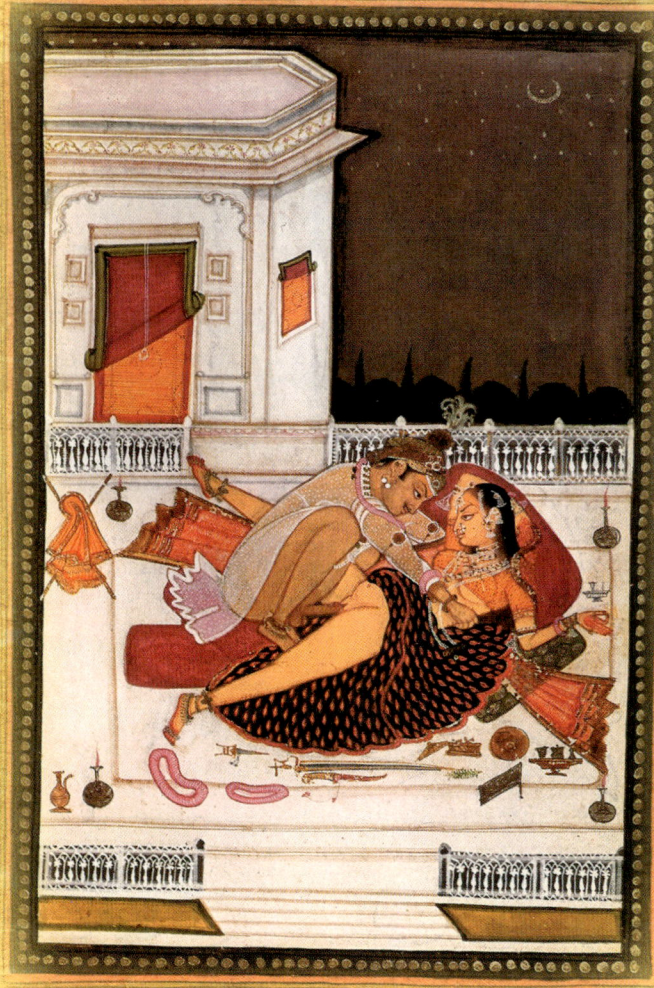

criticizing your size, shape, or smell. It's time to practice unconditional love with this most sacred part of your body.

The Thunderbolt

Okay, guys, now it's your turn. Vatsyayana uses the word *lingam* for "penis." It's a term commonly used in Tantric literature as well. However, in my experience coaching and teaching, I find that many people feel a little uncomfortable with this word. There seems to be something, well, rather *soft* about it. It seems to miss the mark a bit in conveying powerful masculine presence. So I use the word *vajra*, which means "thunderbolt." Vajra is a powerful term in Sanskrit that has a wealth of meanings, including the connotation of king, and it is the name of a very sacred ritual object. So with all due respect to Vatsyayana, I use the word *vajra* in this book.

Just like women, men can carry the same kind of shame and anxiety about their vajra and can be relentlessly critical about how it looks and performs. The same messages to women above apply here for men. Practice unconditional love and acceptance, appreciating all that your vajra does for you (and your partner). It is a sacred tool of your virility that you use to penetrate your beloved with your love, passion, and life force energy. Women love that about you and your vajra.

different? Have you had a chat with your yoni lately about what she wants and needs? Or do you, her owner, boss her around all the time and make all the decisions? If you actually shut up and really listen, it's likely that she has a thing or two to say about who she is and how she wants to be treated. I tell the young girls in my Teen Shakti Rising workshops, "Don't let anyone on, in, or around your sacred temple space who doesn't know how to properly behave in a place of worship." And it must begin with you respecting and honoring yourself. No more denigrating comments or internal dialogue

Other Terms

Here are some other new words for your anatomy that you'll find commonly used throughout this book. I like the term *deva mani* for a man's jewels/balls/gonads. For anus, I use the term *rosetta* (if you think about it, it does look a little like a rose). And for the clitoris, I use the word *pearl*. The G-spot was named after a gynecologist who supposedly "discovered" it, although Tantric masters have spoken of the "sacred spot" for centuries. Both men and women have a sacred spot, which is the term I prefer to use. Try on these new words during lovemaking or make up your own. It can also be fun to give your yoni or vajra a personal name as well. Be open to the perfect name presenting itself.

MAKE IT WORK FOR YOU

If you're single or partnered with someone who's currently not interested in exploring these realms with you, commit to being your own Kama Sutra lover first. Frankly, that's the very best place to begin, even if you do have a willing partner. It's delightful to share sensuality with another human being, but the job of awakening your sexuality is *yours*, not your partner's. Practice self-pleasuring for the sake of expanding and learning about your own orgasmic energy. Pamper your body as a way to heighten your sensual responsiveness. You can even explore many of the Kama Sutra postures on your own. Or you can visualize them with a lover who is likely making his or her way toward you right now. The more you explore your sexual pleasure and give it as an authentic gift to yourself, the more attractive you will naturally be to others.

Also, if you are gay, lesbian, or bisexual and have picked up this book, much of what you find here can be modified for same-sex couples. Please be creative with the positions and substitute language that will support you in loving each other more fully.

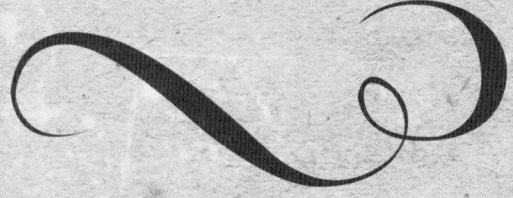

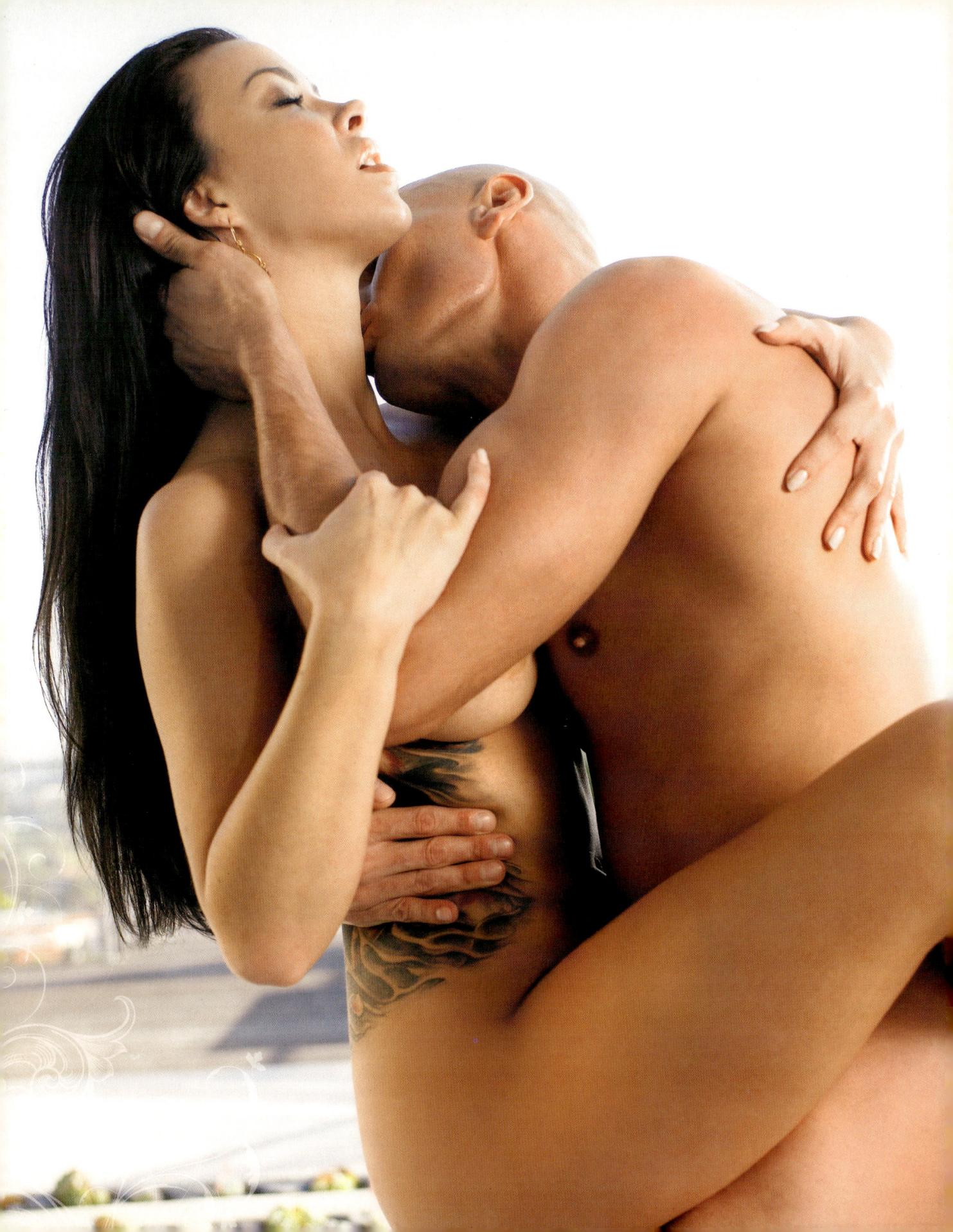

PART II: Kama Sutra Positions

52 OF THE BEST POSITIONS FOR PASSION AND PLEASURE

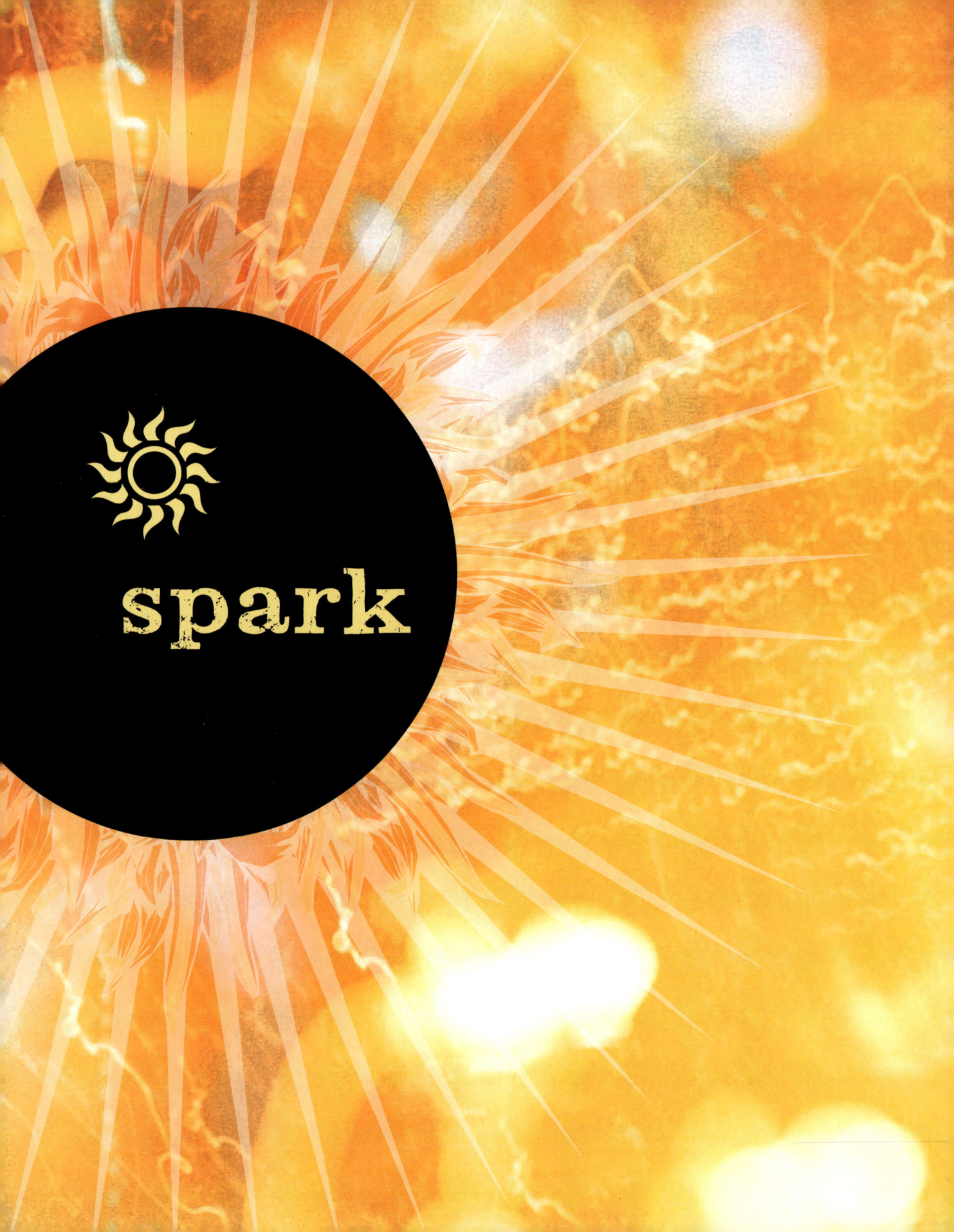

spark

IT ALL BEGINS WITH
A SPARK: A SEDUCTIVE LOOK,
A QUICKENING DEEP IN
THE CORE, THE AWAKENING OF
DESIRE. BEGIN YOUR KAMA SUTRA
JOURNEY WITH THESE POSITIONS
TO WARM YOU UP AND GET
THINGS STARTED. THESE EASY
MOVES, GOOD FOR ALL LOVERS,
WILL BOOST YOUR CONFIDENCE,
GENERATE CLOSENESS,
AND IGNITE PASSION.

1 | RISING SUN

❧ Not Your Basic Missionary Position ❧

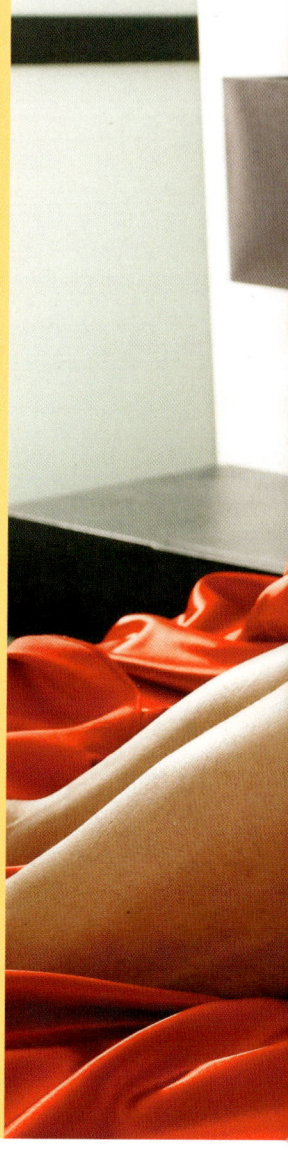

THE STANDARD MISSIONARY POSITION (woman on her back with the man on top facing her) isn't included in our journey of Kama Sutra postures because I figure you've probably got that one down. However, there are many variations on this classic that we'll explore. Some may not look that different on the outside, but what you do on the inside can open up a whole new world of erotic possibilities and sensations.

Unlike the traditional position where the man thrusts and the woman remains passive, in this "Rising Position," as it's called in the Kama Sutra, the man stays still and the woman initiates movement. By rotating on his vajra, she brings both herself and her partner to the dawn of new and fresh pleasures. She also uses his "tool" as an effective means for stimulating various areas in her yoni for healing and awakening.

① The woman lies on her back with her head and upper back supported with pillows. Her knees are bent and open slightly. The man kneels between her legs and supports his weight with his arms outstretched and his back straight above her. He then enters her, but only shallowly and without thrusting.

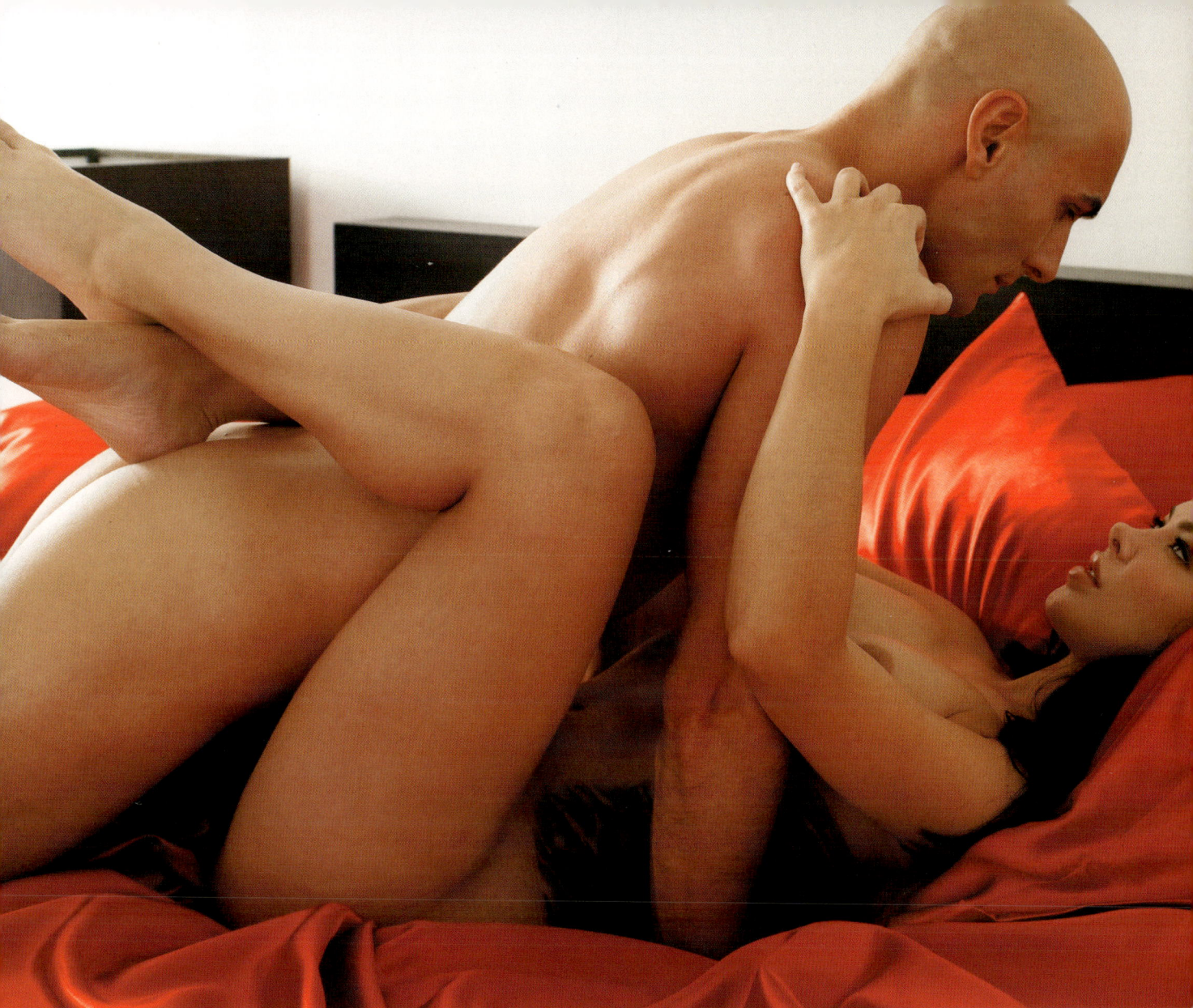

② The woman wraps her legs around him and crosses her ankles behind his back. Reaching up to hold on to him, she then uses both her arms and her legs to vary the angle and depth of penetration.

③ The man remains still while she rotates her pelvis clockwise and then counterclockwise so that she can feel the pressure of his vajra moving along the walls of her yoni, releasing tension and building pleasure. She may also self-pleasure and internally squeeze her yoni muscles to stimulate the rising of their orgasmic energy.

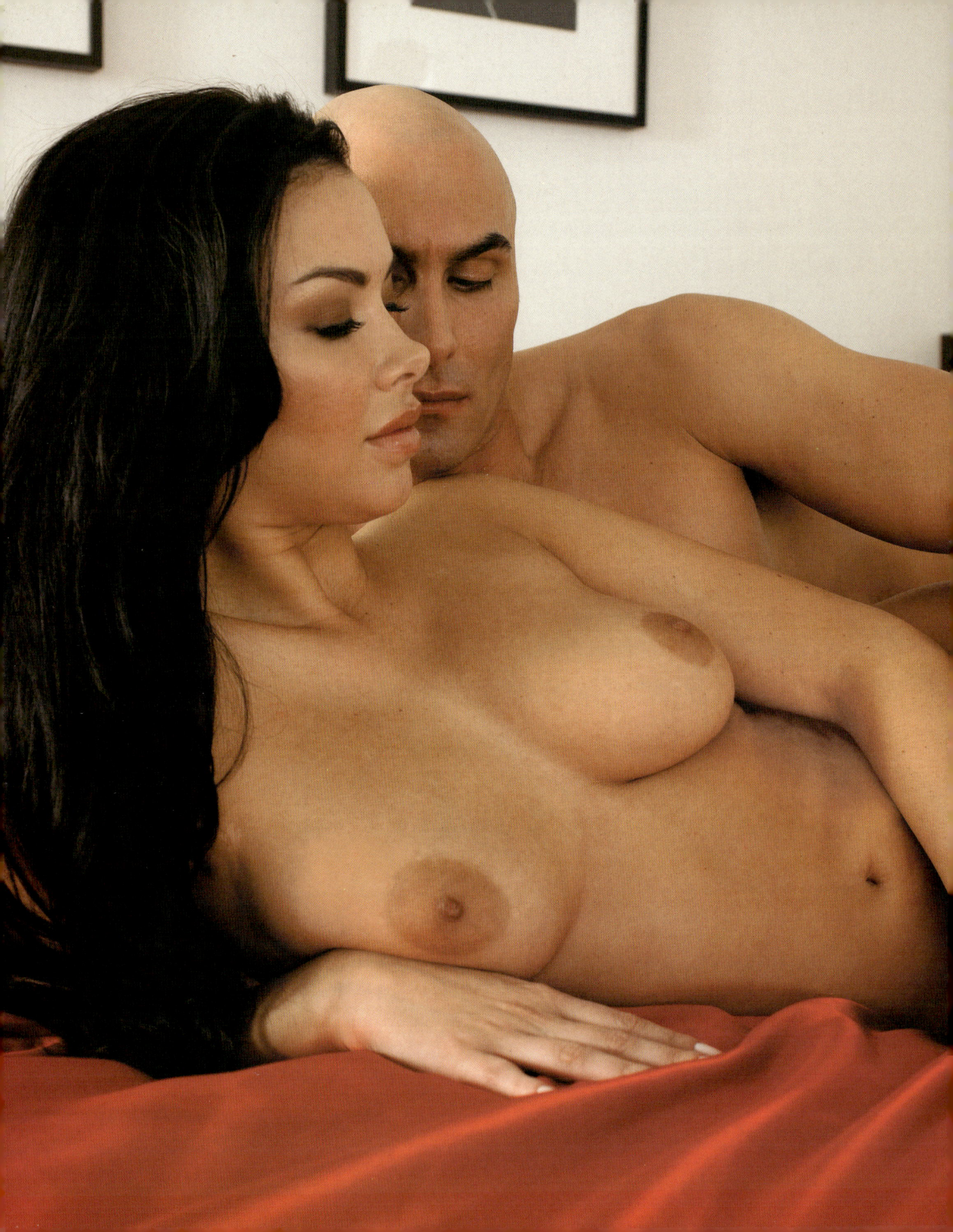

The Importance of Grooming

In the Kama Sutra, Vatsyayana emphasizes the importance of good grooming and bathing prior to lovemaking. His detailed instructions say to eat things that "give fragrance to the mouth," to "bathe daily and anoint the body with oil every other day," and to remove "the sweat of the armpits."

Remember how much time and energy you used to take to get ready for a hot date? Basically, keep doing that. Not to impress the other but as a way of honoring your own body and offering it as a gift to your partner. You can also include bathing and grooming together as part of your lovemaking process rather than in preparation for it.

Make sure you are showered, well manicured and pedicured, and freshly shaved. Shaving the hair of the pubic area can make his deva mani and her yoni irresistible to touch; however, the prickly process of growing the hair back can be a turn-off, so you need to weigh the pros and cons.

Also celebrate the beauty of your body after lovemaking, with your cheeks flushed, your body smelling a little "sex funky," and your messy hair slightly damp with sweat. Hair stylists the world over are trying to capture that look, and they charge a fortune for it.

Come to Your Senses

"Kama includes all enjoyment derived from the five senses," says the Kama Sutra. The best Kama Sutra loving begins well before you get into a sex position. When you take the time to enliven all your senses, you heighten your body's responsiveness and turn on the receptors for ecstasy. Remember that as you work joyfully side by side to prepare your love nest and gather the items that will most delight your senses, you're already engaged in lovemaking.

First things first—get rid of the clutter: the "stuff," anything work-related, the stacks of books, magazines, and mail. Box it up, throw or give it away; get it out of your sacred lovemaking space. Once you have a clean slate, add in colors, objects, and sensual images—anything that makes your space visually beautiful. It's best not to have a TV or computer in your temple space, but if you insist, cover it up.

Use flowers, incense, fragrant candles, or essential oils to add perfume to the air and delight your sense of smell. Choose music for the mood, listen to twinkling wind chimes, moan and talk sexy in your lover's ear. Engage your taste buds with sweet, sour, and salty treats. Suck on slippery mangoes, lick chocolate sauce off her nipple, or give him a sip of fine port—from your mouth. Ignite your tactile senses with feathers, furs, velvet, silks, and satins. And don't forget the edgier delights of scratching, pinching, spanking, and biting.

2 | THE PUMA

{ Hugging His Vajra in Close }

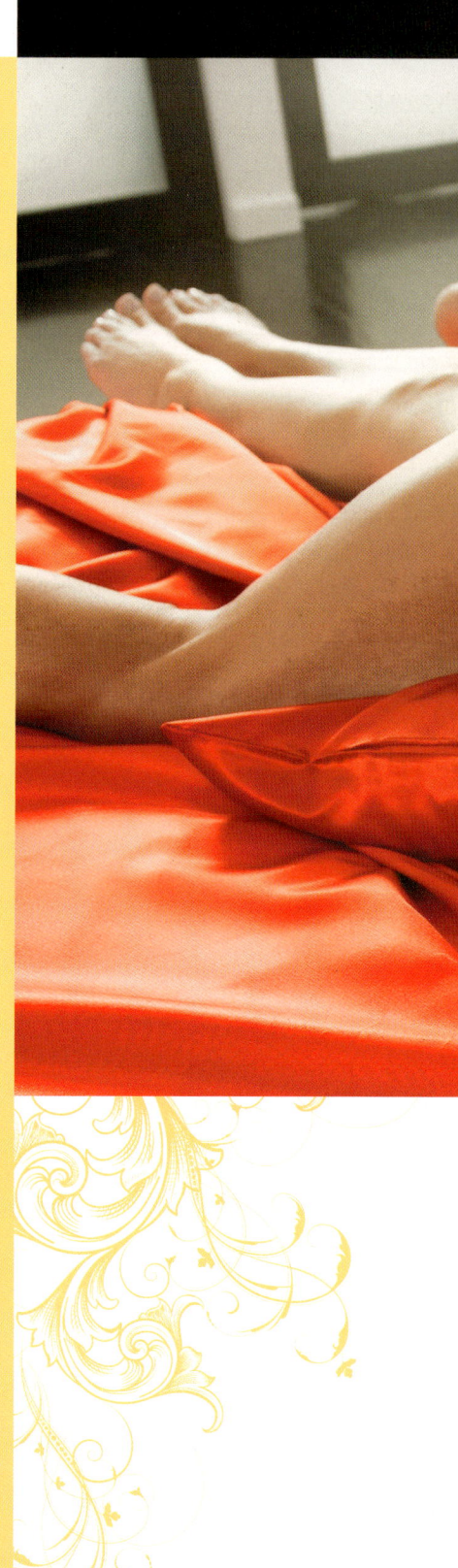

IN THE PUMA, another missionary variation, the woman's legs are pressed together, offering greater stimulation of her outer lips and clitoris. He enjoys the sensation of his vajra being fully hugged between her legs. The position leaves her hands free to roam where they please: caressing his chest, stimulating his nipples or her own, pleasuring her pearl.

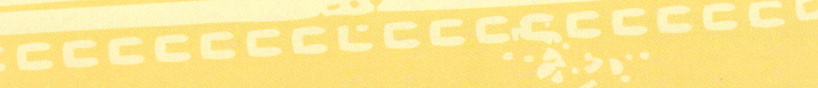

"A man does not succeed either by implicitly following the inclination of a girl, or by wholly opposing her, and he should therefore adopt a middle course. He who knows how to make himself beloved by women, as well as to increase their honor and create confidence in them, this man becomes an object of their love."

—*Mallinaga Vatsyayana*

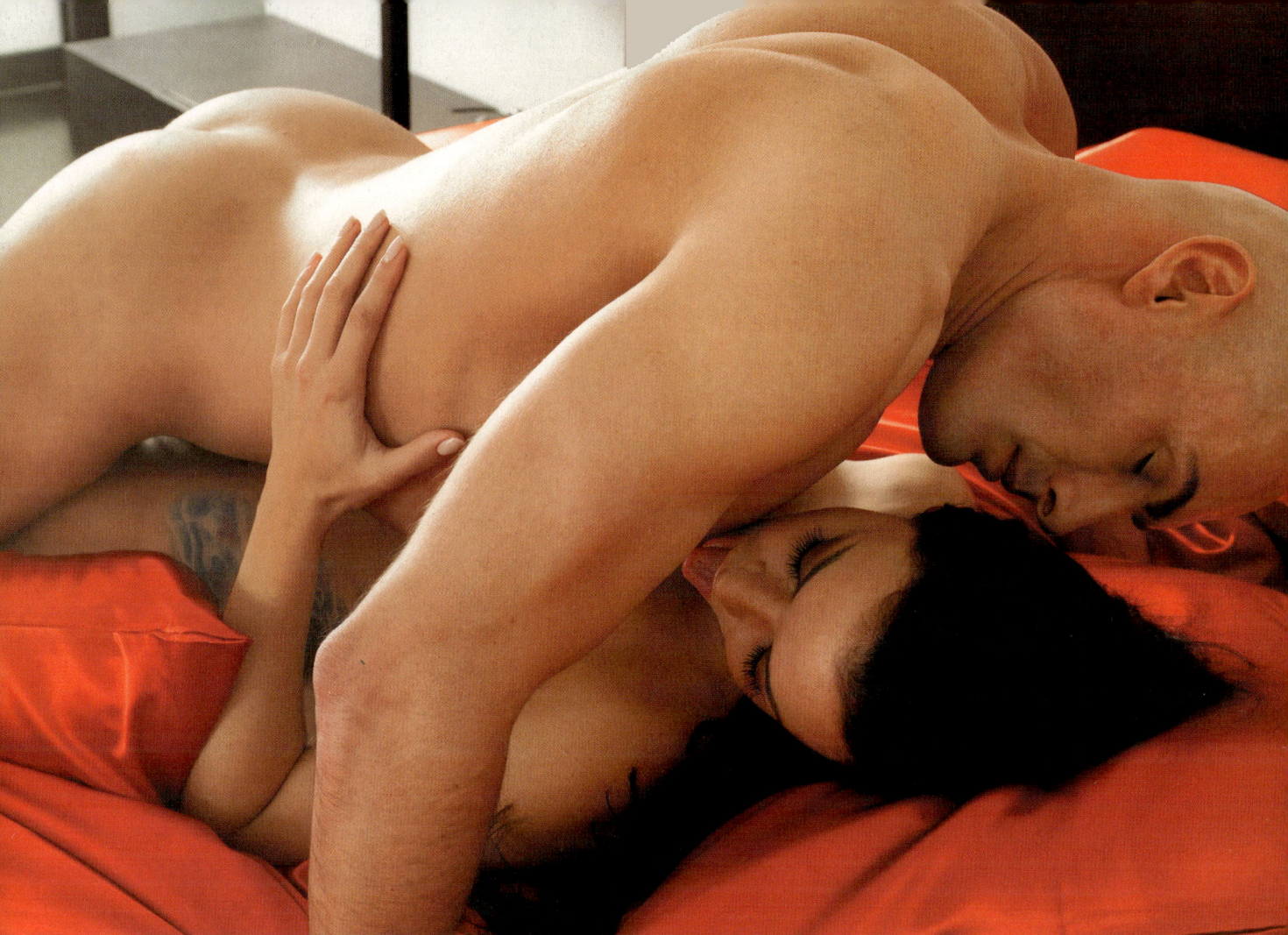

① The man enters the woman lying on her back in the traditional missionary style with her knees open to the side.

② The man leans to one side and then to the other to assist the woman in bringing her legs together inside his. Her legs are straight down and pressed together, grasping his vajra. His thighs are now on the outside of hers, and he supports the weight of his upper body with his arms outstretched alongside her. By tilting her pelvis forward (or placing a pillow under her butt), the woman may be able to enjoy clitoral stimulation each time her puma lunges toward her.

③ Although not all men enjoy nipple stimulation, it can be highly erotic and even orgasmic for some. With a pillow propped up behind her head, the woman can suck on his nipples to pleasure him and assist them both in drawing sexual energy up from the pelvis to the higher chakras (energy centers in the body). He may also be able to hold her head to his chest with one arm as he supports his weight with the other.

3 YAWNING OPEN

{ Wide Open Surrender }

FAR FROM PUTTING either of you to sleep, the Yawning Open position in the Kama Sutra refers to the woman being wide awake and open. By lying on her back with her legs pointing up to the sky, the woman can experience a concentration of sexual energy as the blood flows to her pelvis. Women can be turned on by the erotic act of full surrender this position demands, while most men will experience her complete openness as a powerful aphrodisiac.

① The Yawning Open position starts with the woman lying on her back with her legs wide open in a V shape. Place a few firm pillows under her hips so that the mound of her yoni is raised and open, like a jewel on display. The man positions himself between her legs and takes this opportunity to stroke her, admire her body, and arouse her with his hands, tongue, and words of love. When you are both ready, she can bend her legs and tilt her pelvis to help him enter her as he kneels before her.

② She then straightens her legs and lifts them up to the sky so that they are perpendicular to her body as she opens them wide in a V shape. By pointing her toes, the woman can activate stronger energy in her legs, visualizing life force streaming into her toes, down her legs, and into her sacred well, where she nourishes herself and her man. The man provides the movement in this posture, while the woman receives. It's also an ideal position for her to stimulate her clitoris as she rides the waves of orgasm with her beloved.

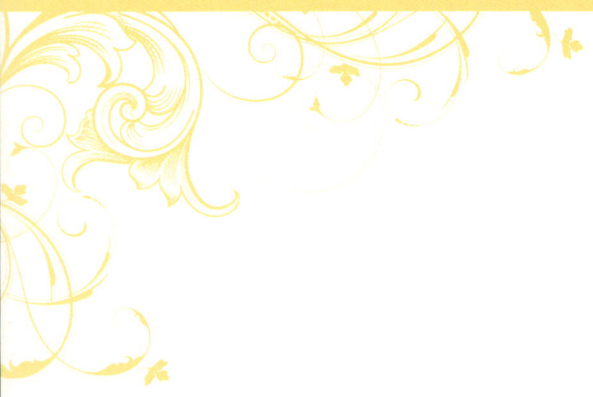

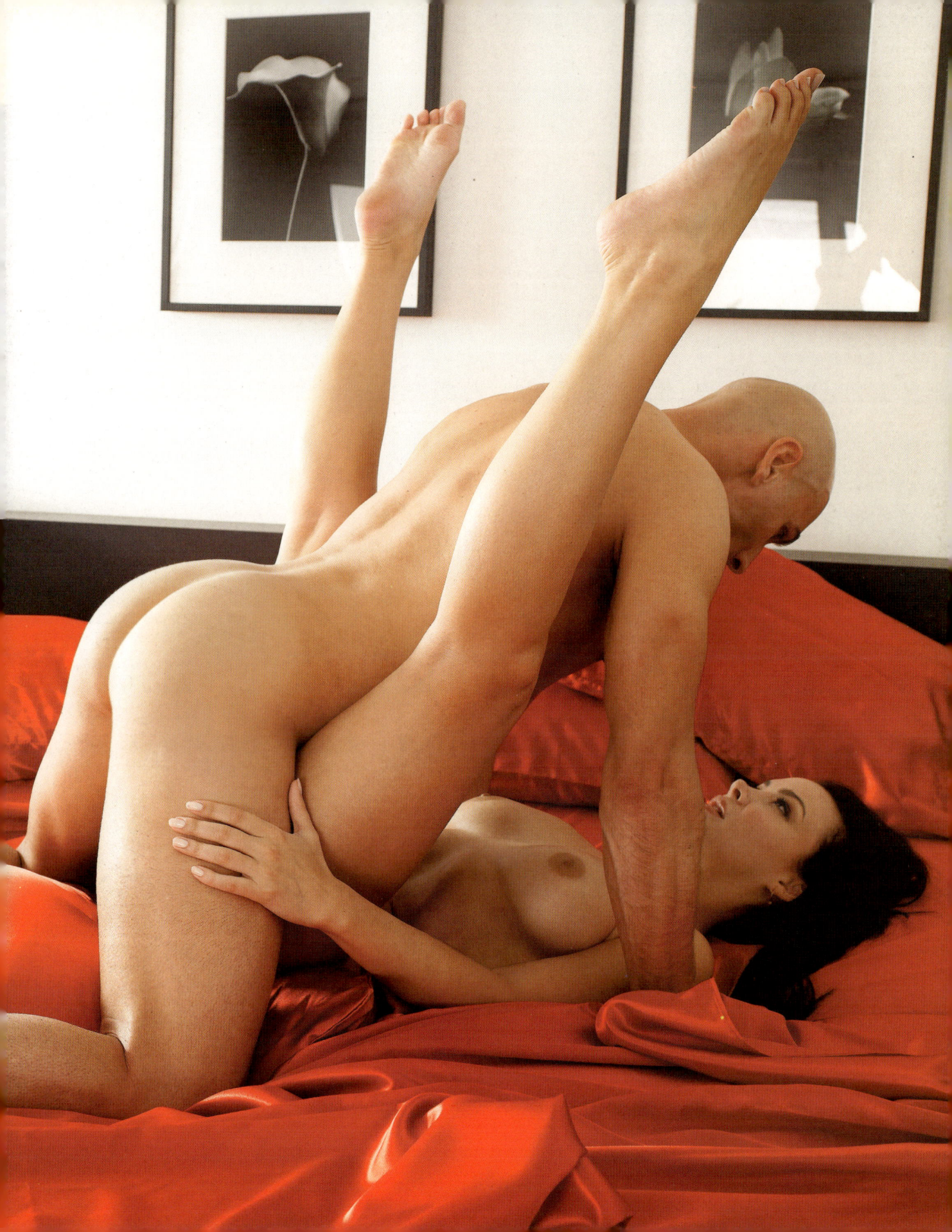

4 | CLIMBING A TREE

{ Slithering Sensually Up His Trunk }

THE ART OF EMBRACING was a serious study in the original Kama Sutra text, with Vatsyayana describing detailed variations called for in different situations. In this classic embrace, the woman appears to be climbing up the trunk of her man to reach his mouth for a kiss. It can be used to generate intimacy and can move into a posture of sexual union as well.

① The man begins by standing with his feet slightly apart and planted on a firm surface as if he were a tree rooted to the earth. The woman approaches him and places her feet on top of his, balancing her weight evenly and wrapping her arms around him for added support. In this gesture of devotion, a woman "leaves the earth" and surrenders to her man's strength as he holds and cares for her.

② As you embrace more closely and kiss each other's hungry mouths, the woman shifts her weight to one foot and "climbs" higher up her man with her other leg. Depending on her height and strength, she may be able to hook her bent leg around her man and squeeze him more tightly to her. Alternately, he can assist her by reaching down to support her bent leg with his opposite arm. If intercourse is desired, she can rock her pelvis back to assist him in entering her. With his hand supporting her leg, he can move her rhythmically as you both climb to the heights of pleasure.

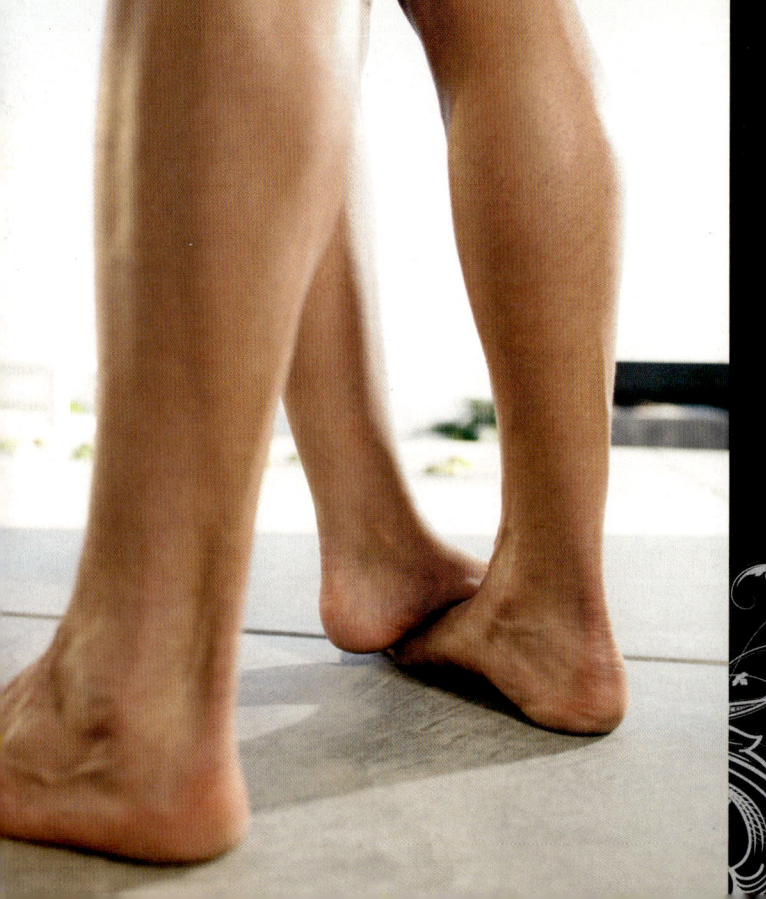

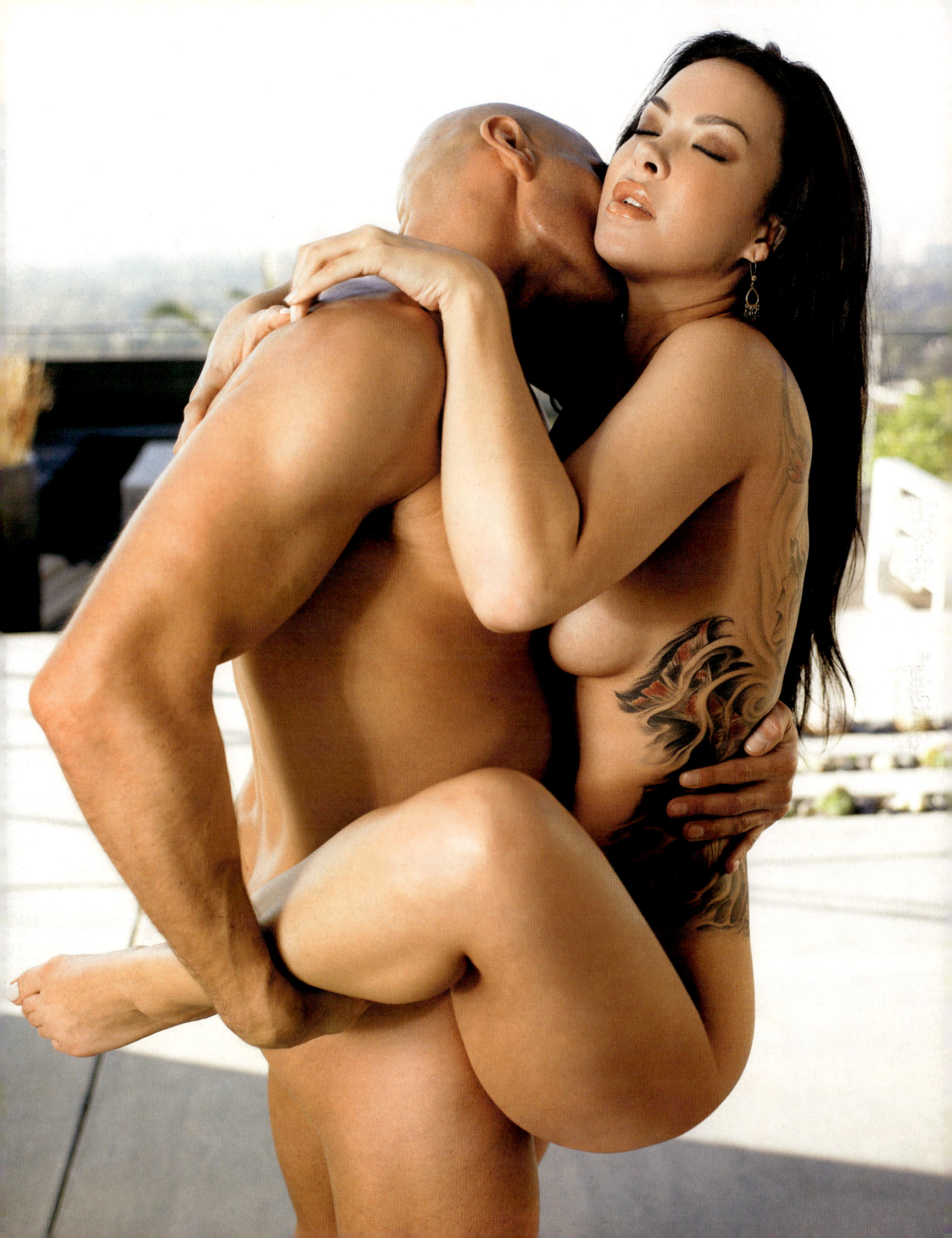

5 | NAMASTÉ

{ *Honoring Creates Profound Opening* }

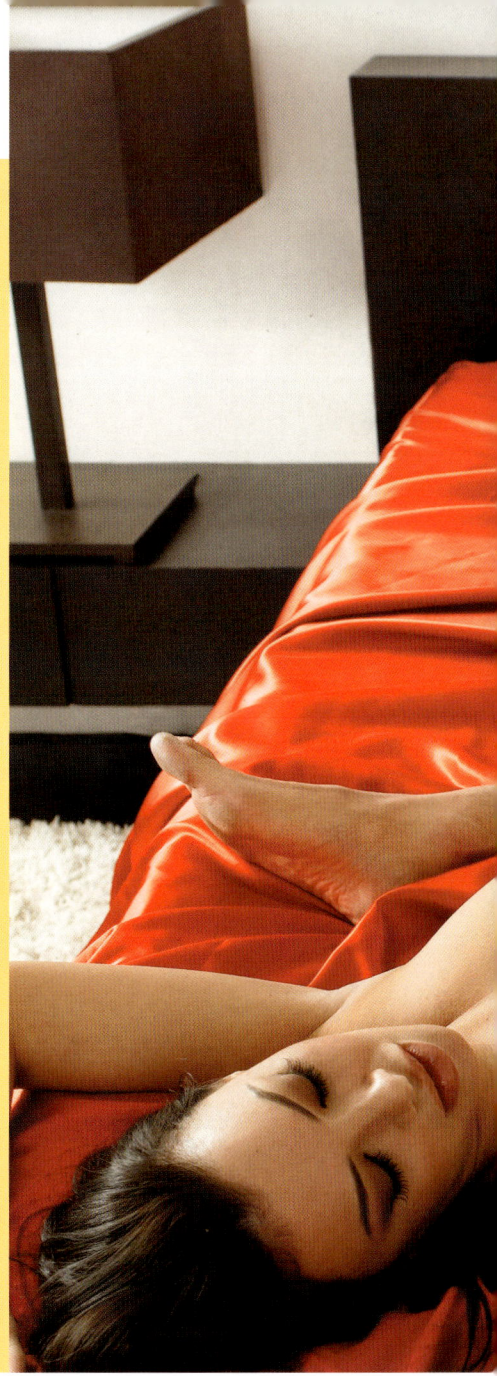

NAMASTÉ (pronounced NA-ma-stay) is a Sanskrit word that means "the divine essence in me bows to and honors the divine essence in you; when I am in that place in me and you are in that place in you, we are one." In this posture, the sacred masculine in him honors the sacred feminine in her. A wise man doesn't have to be a Tantric master to know that when he honors the goddess in his woman, she often overflows with gifts in return.

If used before intercourse, this position is a powerful way to set the tone for a deeper feeling of intimacy. During sex, it's a good way to move the sexual energy from the pelvis to the higher chakra energy centers in the body, for more expansive orgasms. It's perhaps most ideal after orgasm as a way to show gratitude for her opening her body and soul. Don't be surprised if this gesture brings tears of joy to the woman, who may have never been honored in this way before.

① The woman lies on her back with her knees gently open, fully surrendered. He sits upright between her legs so that their genitals are pressed together or he is inside her. She places one hand on his leg in loving connection and raises her other arm over her head to fully open her heart to receive his blessing.

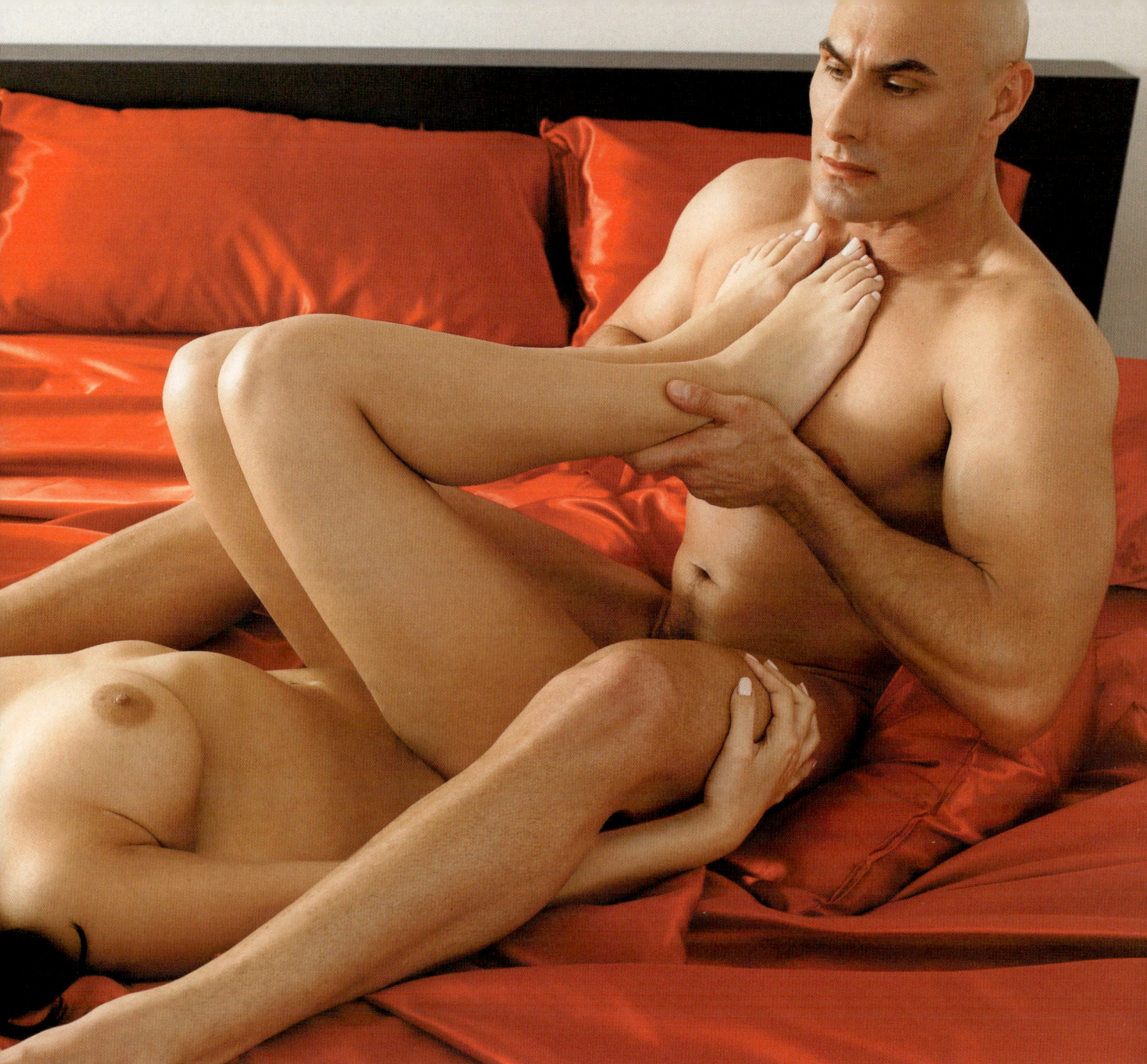

② He closes his eyes and takes a few breaths to prepare himself, entering into a state of devotion. When he's ready, he looks into her eyes and gently lifts her feet with both hands and holds them to his heart. With his eyes, he silently conveys to her how much she touches him. He then brings her feet to his lips and kisses them.

③ Next he touches her feet to the intuitive power point between his brows. Finally, he rests the soles of her feet on his forehead with her toes reaching toward the crown of his head. This final gesture acknowledges the power she has to bring him to closer to heaven. To close, he speaks the word "Namasté" to her from his heart. The woman can also perform this ritual for her man.

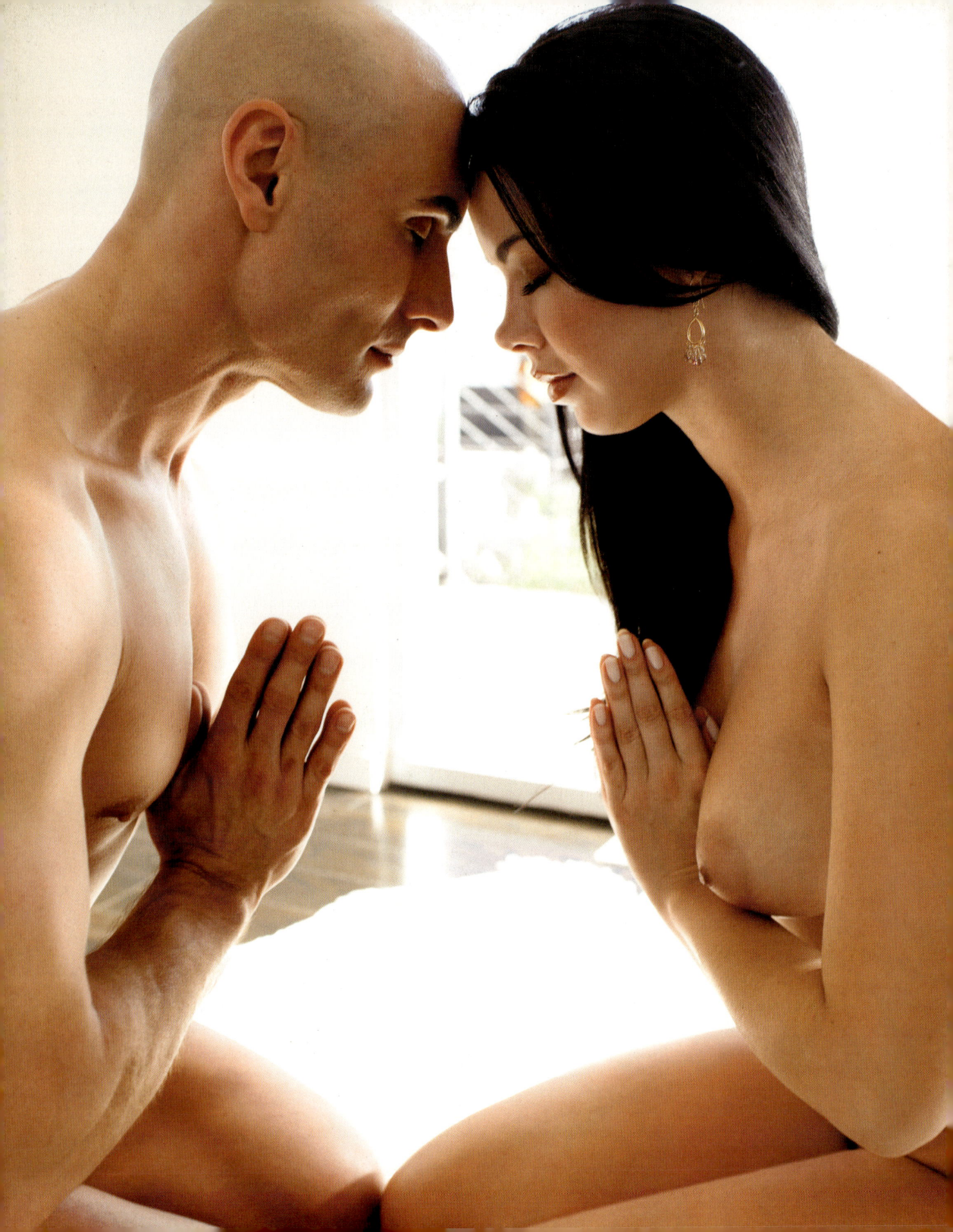

Start with the Heart

The Heart Salutation is an ancient but simple yogic ritual that can have a dramatic effect on your lovemaking. It only takes a few moments, and it works like magic to get you present, align mind-body-soul, and bring you into harmony with yourself and your partner either before or after sex. Perhaps most importantly, it telegraphs a message to the sacred realms, calling in blessings on your lovemaking and releasing the intention that the ecstasy generated by your union serve the highest and greatest good of all.

① Begin by sitting with your knees together, your butt resting on your feet on a soft, cushioned surface (a fluffy sheepskin is ideal), facing each other knee to knee. Slowly expand your breathing. Take several moments to relax, looking deeply into each other's eyes. See beyond his or her personality and come into resonance with the god or goddess that resides deep within, feeling that same divinity inside you. Bring your hands together in a prayer position and touch your fingertips to the ground between your knees. Breathe in unison with your partner.

② On an inhalation, imagine drawing the earth energy up as you lift your hands to your heart and sit upright. Continue the inhalation until you can hold no more, and stay in constant eye contact with your partner.

③ As you exhale, bow forward slowly until you gently come to rest your forehead against your beloved's. Close your eyes and take two deep breaths together, feeling the energy moving between the sacred point between your eyebrows known as the Third Eye, or center of inner vision.

④ At the conclusion of the second connected forehead breath, inhale deeply as you open your eyes, look at your partner, and sit back again on your heels with your hands still resting against your heart.

⑤ As you exhale, drop your hands back down to the earth, returning the energy and completing the circle.

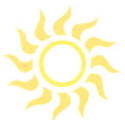

6 | REUNION

{ The Delicious Anticipation of Togetherness }

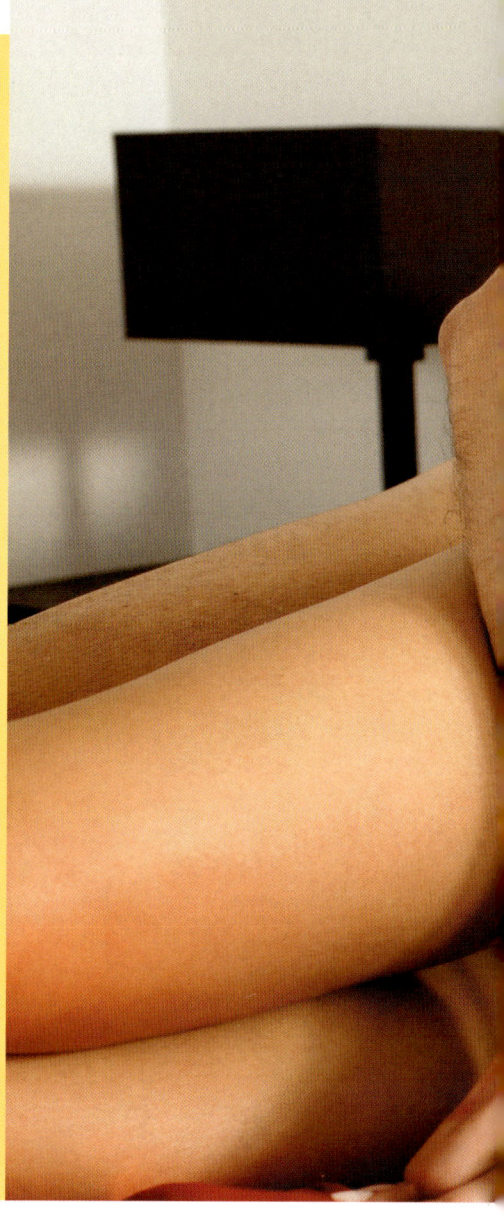

THE BODY PROCESSES information differently than the mind, so even if you and your lover understand that a period of separation has ended, your body may be still holding on to sadness or confusion that needs to be released so you can open fully to each other again. Whether the separation was due to travel, an emotional upset, or just the busyness of life keeping you apart, this posture is an effective way to bypass the mind, clear that energy from the body, and spark your connection again. The posture involves a bit of role-playing, so have fun with it.

① The woman begins by positioning herself on the bed with her back to the entrance of the room, leaning on her side with her legs and knees together and her body upright, resting on an outstretched arm. Although facing away from the door, she tilts her ear toward the entrance as if listening for the sound of her lover returning. The man approaches slowly and quietly, taking some time to appreciate his beloved poised and waiting for him. Before joining

her, the man takes several breaths loud enough for his beloved to hear so you can both relish the anticipation of being reunited.

② The man approaches the woman very slowly from behind and touches her tenderly on her feet. At this point, she can turn to him and make eye contact, watching him as he slowly massages her feet and then caresses her calves, knees, and thighs. As his

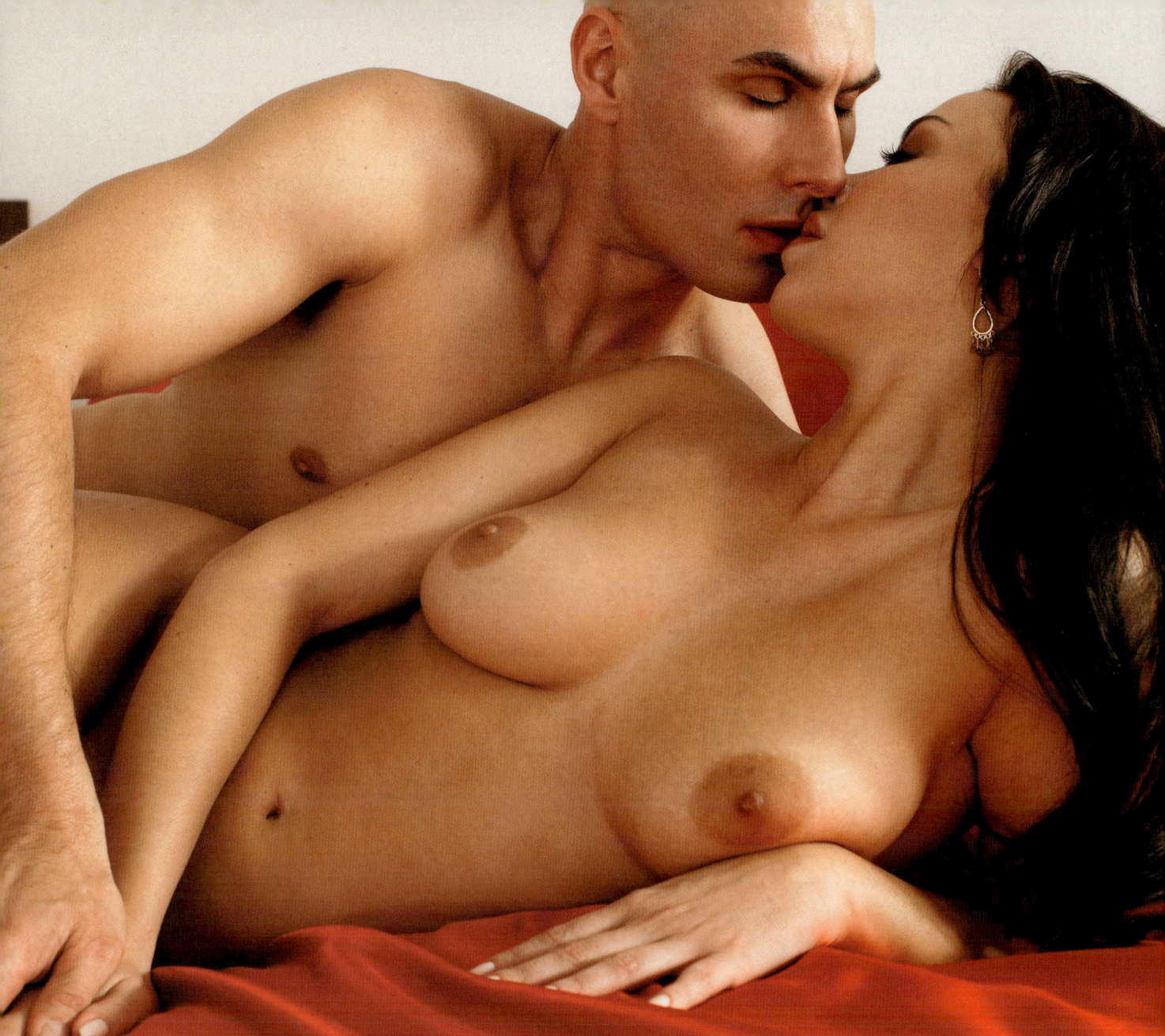

touch moves up her body to her butt, belly, breasts, and shoulders, she will likely begin to melt into his body behind her, delighting in his strength and the feeling of his protective embrace.

③ She can then kiss him deeply. As the passion builds, he will eventually press his entire body against the back of hers. She will open her legs and tilt her hips toward him to invite him to enter her. From here, you

move in ecstasy together as the man alternates between shallow and deep thrusting. In this way, you celebrate your orgasmic union, dispelling any distance between you. After climaxing, both partners stay in this position together, "spooning" for as long as possible, allowing the orgasmic energy to work its magical healing.

7 SESAME AND RICE

{ The Joy of Intertwined Connection }

IN ANOTHER of the classic Kama Sutra embraces, the lovers in this position are so intertwined that it would be as difficult as separating sesame and rice to pull them apart. A beautiful embrace for beginning or ending a lovemaking session, it is also conducive for deeply bonding intercourse. By facing each other fully, you can kiss passionately or transmit your love to one another through your eyes. In an embrace like this, we forget separation and merge together as one.

① Begin by lying down, facing each other with your knees gently touching and your arms loosely around one another. Look deeply into each other's eyes, soul gaze and breathe in harmony.

② Begin kissing one another, gently at first with little nibbles and plenty of pauses. Take turns receiving kisses passively, then giving.

③ As the sexual energy begins to build, press your bodies closer together. Wrap your arms more firmly around each other. The woman lifts her uppermost leg up and over the man's hip. As she does so, he slides his uppermost leg between her legs and rests his thigh against her open yoni (or enters her if desired). Intertwine your outstretched legs and enjoy the delicious closeness of your bodies.

Soul Gazing

The eyes are a "window to the soul." We trust people who make good eye contact. New lovers can't take their eyes off each other; time seems to stand still. When we look deeply into the eyes of our partner, we experience heart-opening intimacy that paves the way for ecstatic lovemaking.

Practice sitting across from your Beloved and simply be. Breathe deeply and slowly, gazing into your lover's eyes (pick one side so your eyes aren't darting). You don't have to smile or take care of them; just relax your face. When thoughts intrude, let them go like clouds floating by.

Keep bringing yourself back to your breath and being fully present with your partner. Although the first few minutes may feel awkward (or induce a fit of laughter), soon you will feel calm and peaceful. The longer you soul gaze with your partner, the more their essence will be revealed to you. You stop seeing the personality and begin to discern the divine being that resides within them—the very same spark of God-Goddess that looks through your eyes. When you move into lovemaking from this space, you open the door for the kind of transcendent, ecstatic experiences that mystics have been writing about for centuries.

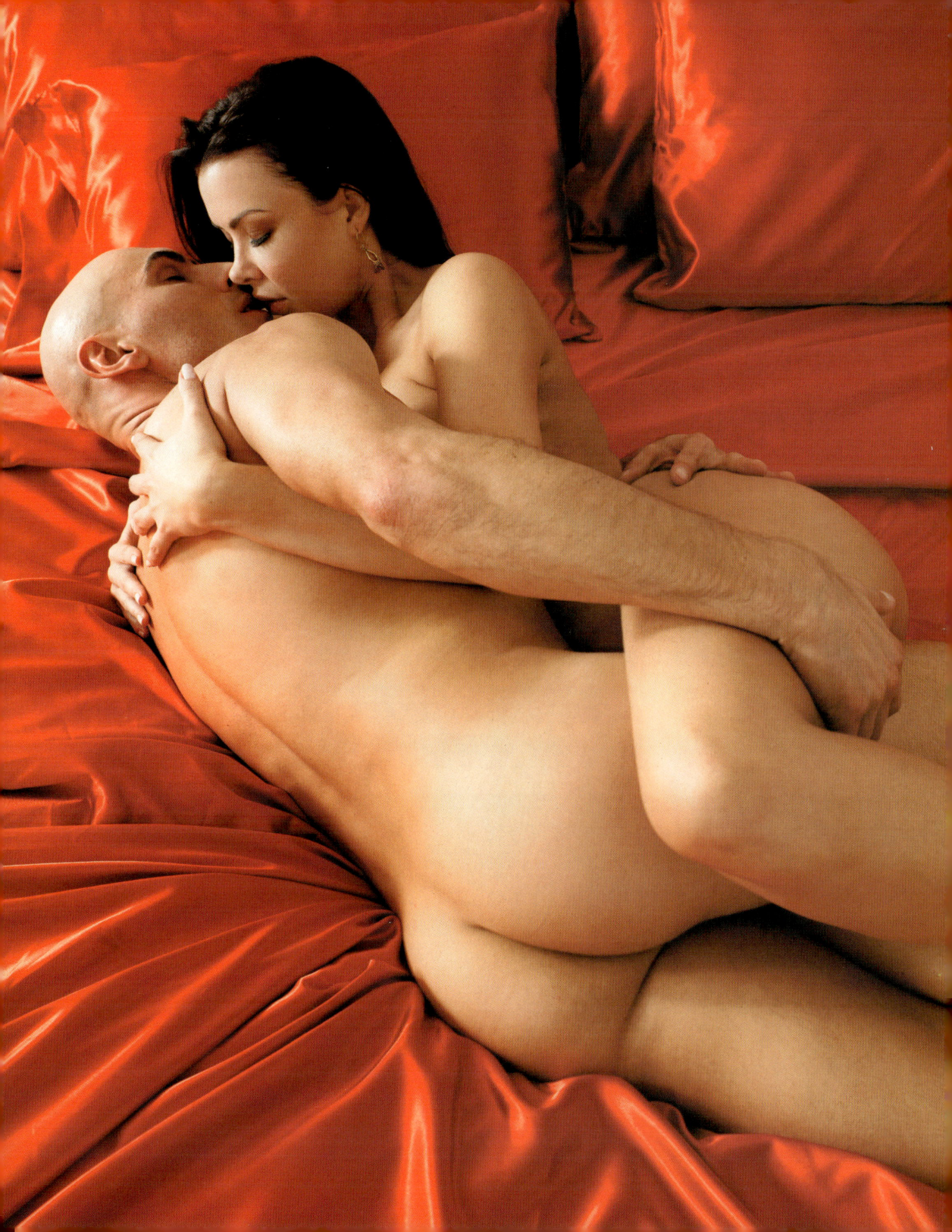

8

BOW AND ARROW

❧ *More Than Just Spooning* ❧

ALTHOUGH THIS POSITION can be done anytime, it's particularly delicious coming out of sleep, either for early morning lovemaking or when passion quickens in the middle of the night. Because it begins in a classic spooning position, it's an easy position to move into when cuddling sparks the flame of desire.

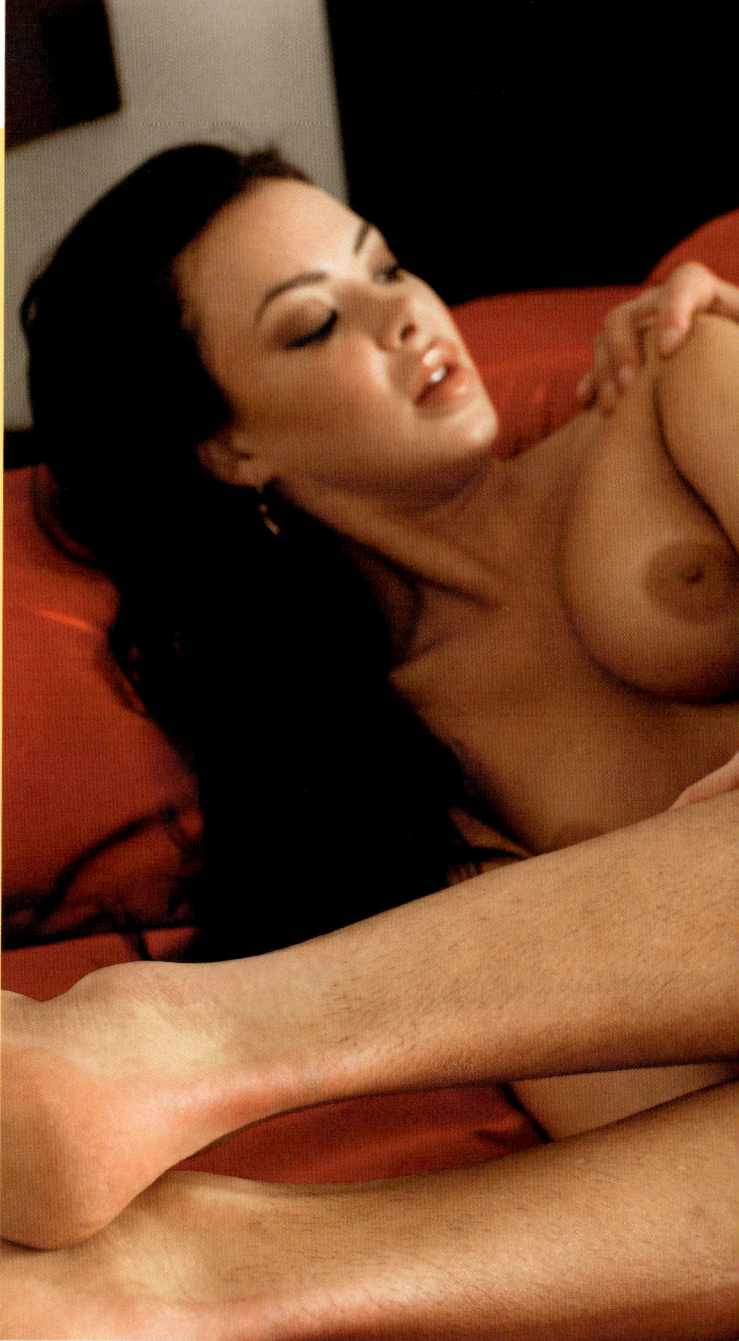

① The woman lies on her side with the man spooning her from behind. As your arousal builds, the man can either place his erection "up" in the cleft of her butt or place it between her thighs so that it stimulates the outside lips of her yoni until she is ready for penetration.

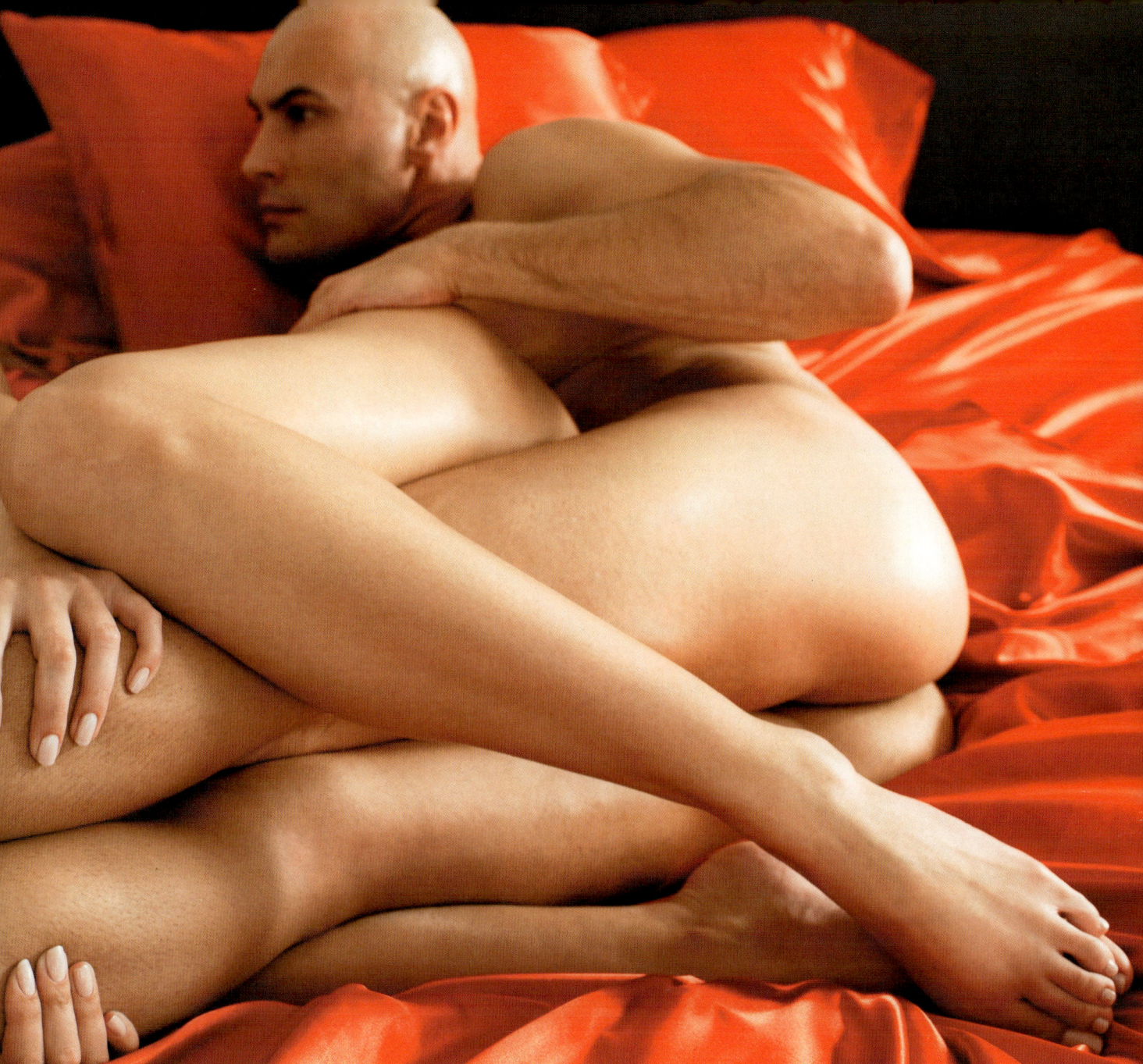

② He then parts her legs with his knees and enters her, holding her around the shoulders in order to move more deeply and rhythmically inside her. She places her top leg over his upper leg and squeezes him more closely to her.

③ She then reaches down toward his feet and grasps his ankles or lower legs firmly. She is now perpendicular to him, becoming the "arrow" inside the curved "bow" shape of his body. Both of you move together in this position. She pulls on his legs for leverage as she rocks her pelvis into him, and he thrusts into her by pulling her hips toward him. Eventually, you may find that you both have to let that arrow fly to its target.

9 | STAR FLOWER

{ Crisscross into a Star }

THE NAME OF THIS BEAUTIFUL POSE comes from the flowerlike opening of the lovers as they intertwine in a crisscross star-shaped pattern. It is an erotically stimulating position as well as a powerful restorative posture after climaxing. It allows lovers to stay connected at the root chakra, or perineum, where the "X" of their bodies generates powerful union.

At the same time, it reinforces your individual wholeness as you stretch apart from one another.

① The man sits upright with his legs slightly apart, his left leg out straight and his right knee bent with his right foot flat on the bed or floor. He supports his weight on his arms, which are outstretched behind him. The woman sits diagonally on top of him, threading her outstretched left leg under his bent right knee and placing her right leg over his left, her right knee bent with her foot flat on the bed or floor beside him. Like him, she supports herself with her arms stretched out behind her.

② Bring your right hands to rest on one another's right shoulders, creating a starlike pattern with your bodies. As the man enters the woman, you can slowly slide your hands down each other's arms, finding the right tension and holding on to each other to balance and facilitate the most pleasurable movements. Depending on the direction of the "hook" of the man's vajra, you will both feel different sensations depending on whether you are angled to the right or the left. With some practice, you will discover whether one side of the star generates more pleasure for one or both of you.

③ As the passion subsides after orgasm or during a break in lovemaking, maintain eye contact with your lover and slowly loosen your grip on his or her arm. Allow your right hands to slide down each other's arms until you're just touching fingertips, coming down to support yourselves on your opposite elbow and eventually helping each other to lie back fully.

④ In the final expression of this pose, the woman brings her hands together over her head as if to create a halo of starlight, and the man rests his hand palm down on her outstretched leg, grounding her and staying connected. This is a perfect posture for drifting off into blissful slumber with one another.

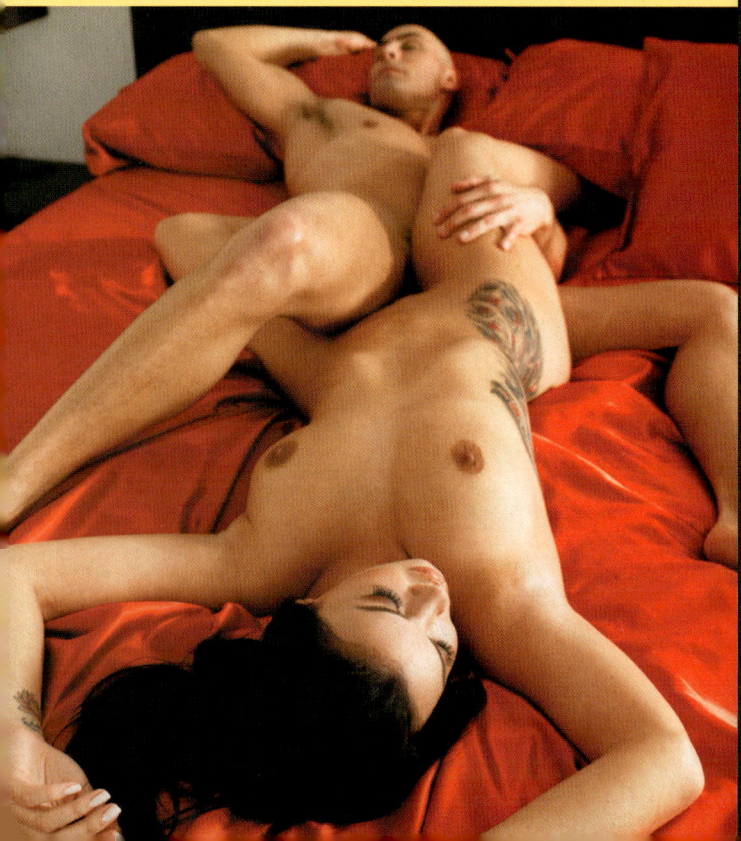

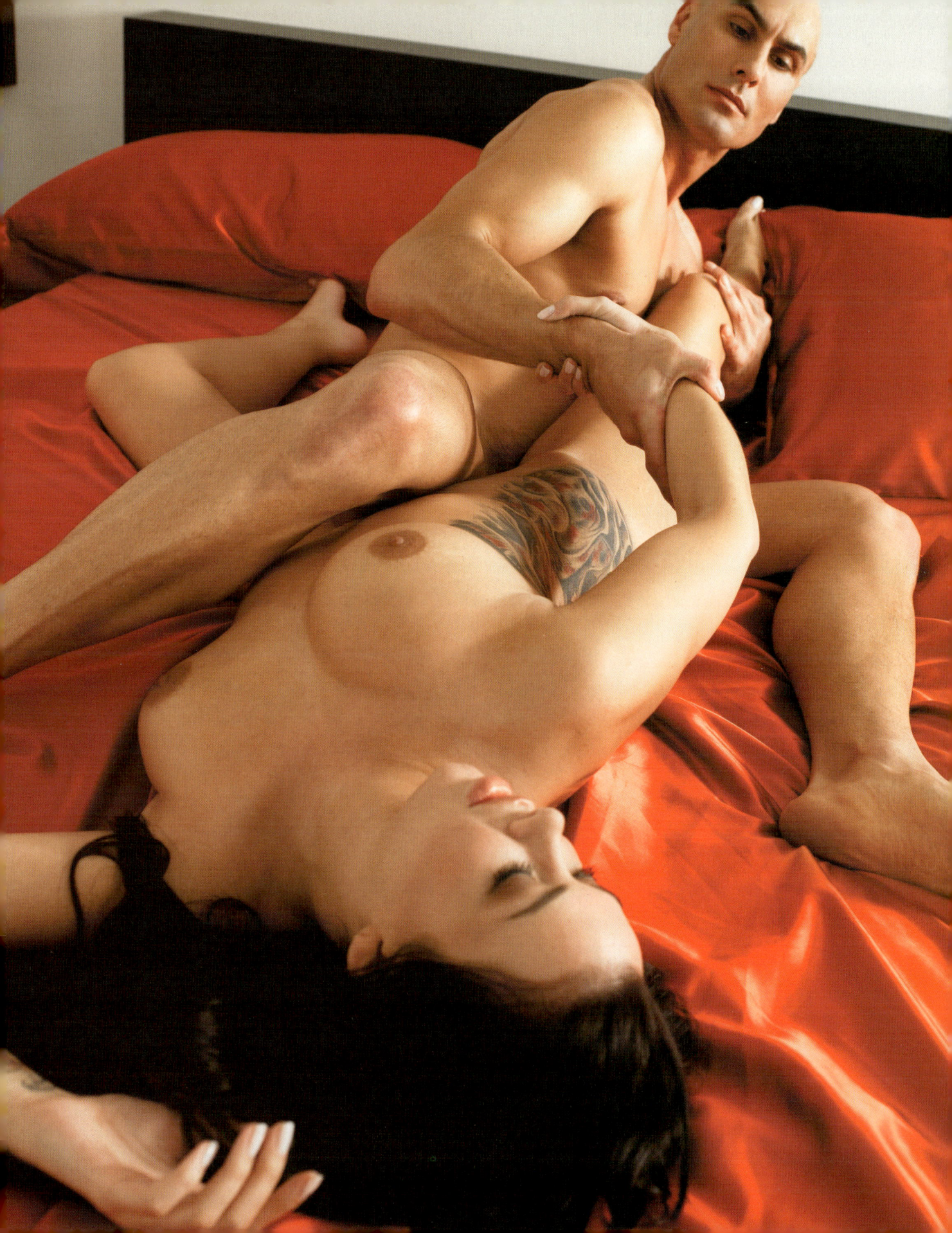

10 | YIN YANG

{ *Opposites United as One* }

IN THIS POSITION, the masculine and feminine are both opposite and united at the same time, just like the classic Eastern symbol of light and dark. This can be a good position for gentle penetration or for taking a break during more vigorous lovemaking. It's also ideal for the afterglow period following orgasm, when it's important to stay connected to your partner so your body can best integrate the sexual energy you just created.

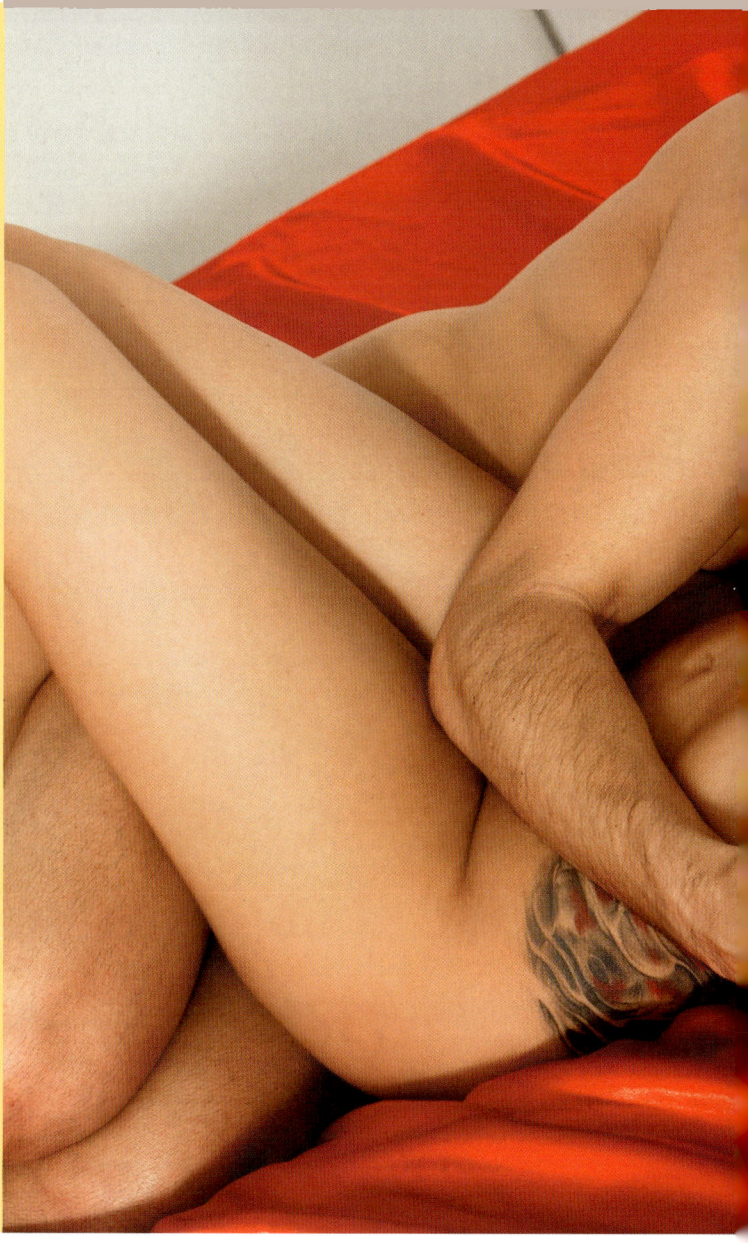

① The woman lies on her back with her arms up, resting alongside her head. This will allow for deeper expansion of her lungs and opening of her heart. Her butt and yoni should be nestled against her man's vajra with her legs gently draped over his hips. The

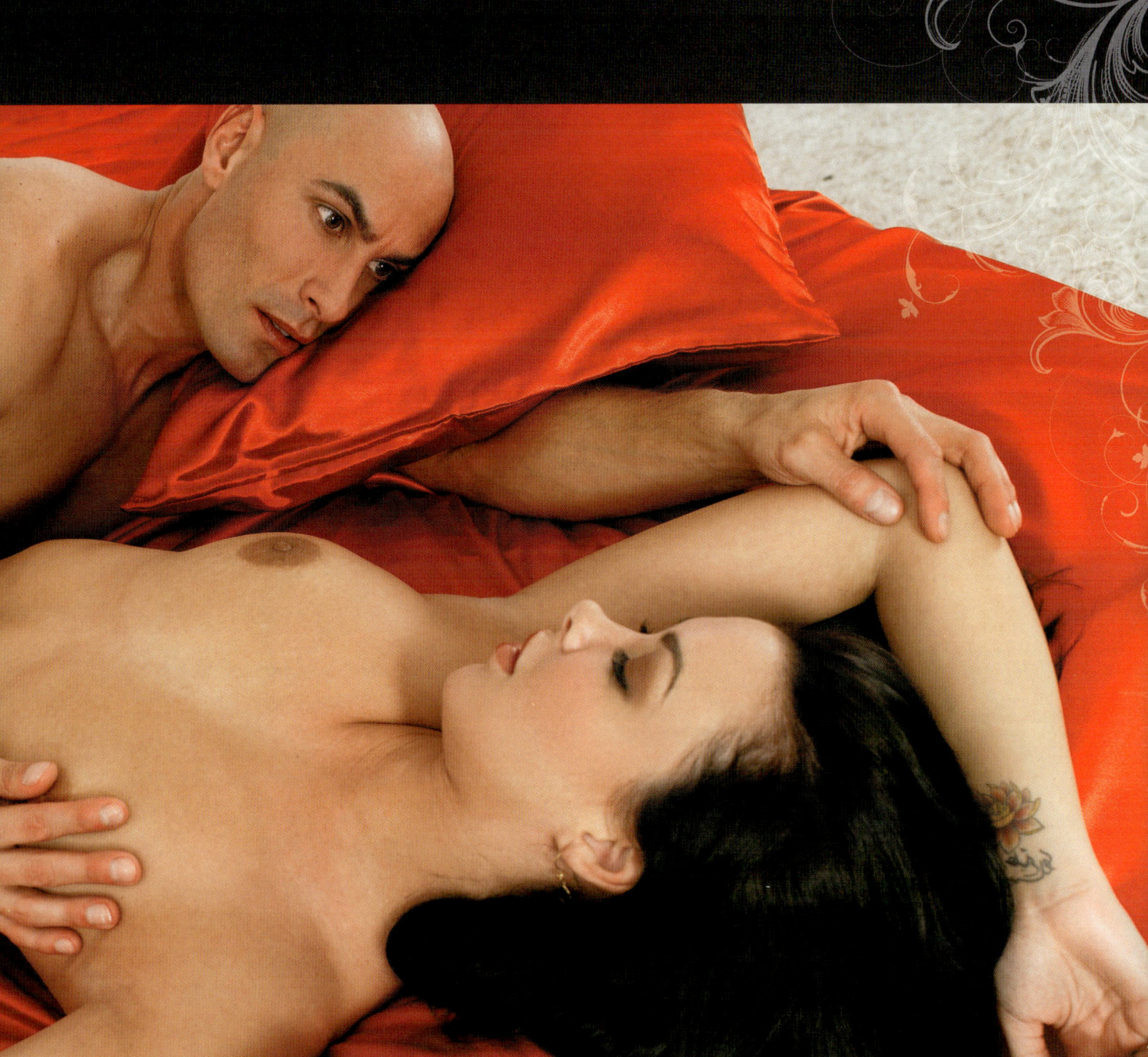

man lies perpendicular to her on his side, with one arm holding her legs on top of him and the other free to caress her breasts or body. A pillow under his head and others propped up behind him will give him the support he needs to fully relax in this posture.

② To invigorate his vajra and create more sexual energy in this position, the woman can use her yoni muscles to squeeze and suck him while you both remain motionless externally. The opposite and united "knot" created by the two pelvises in this position can magnetize sexual energy between you during intercourse. Used before or after lovemaking, this position brings balance to a couple along with a feeling of individual union within.

11 | COCOON

{ Wrapped Up Together in Bliss }

IN THIS DELICIOUS EMBRACE, couples experience a feeling of being cocooned in love and pleasure. The cozy closeness of this position is great for gentle lovemaking, as a warm-up for other positions, or as a cool-down after lovemaking.

"Your sexuality is God's love letter to you, a miracle of biological engineering that could have been devised only by a mind of vast and humorous generosity, a mind that knew the pain and the sense of confinement earthly beings would feel and wanted to make sure you might always have glimpses of heaven."

—*Jalaja Bonheim,*
Aphrodite's Daughters

① The man kneels on both knees and sits back on the soles of his feet, the tops of his feet pressed into the bed. Depending on his knee flexibility, he may be more comfortable with a soft pillow underneath him to raise his hips slightly and take pressure off his knees.

② The woman sits on his lap and wraps her legs around him, touching her feet together behind him. The man should place his vajra "up," whether he is erect or not, so the woman can nuzzle the outer lips of her yoni around him. In this position, you can soul gaze, hold each other closely, stroke each other's backs, and kiss deeply to come into harmony and open yourselves to pleasure.

③ Once fully aroused, the woman can clasp her hands around her lover's neck, press into her feet, and raise herself up in order to take him inside her. She can do so quickly, or she can seductively tease just the tip of his vajra by tilting her pelvis forward so that her yoni makes only subtle contact until you are both begging for deeper penetration.

④ The man supports the woman by holding her around the small of her back. When she is held firmly, she can lean back, hold him around the neck, lift her feet up, and surrender to his trusting embrace. She can adjust the angle of penetration by lifting her legs and rocking back and forth on him. The man uses his pelvis and arms to rock her back and forth, finding a rhythm of ecstasy.

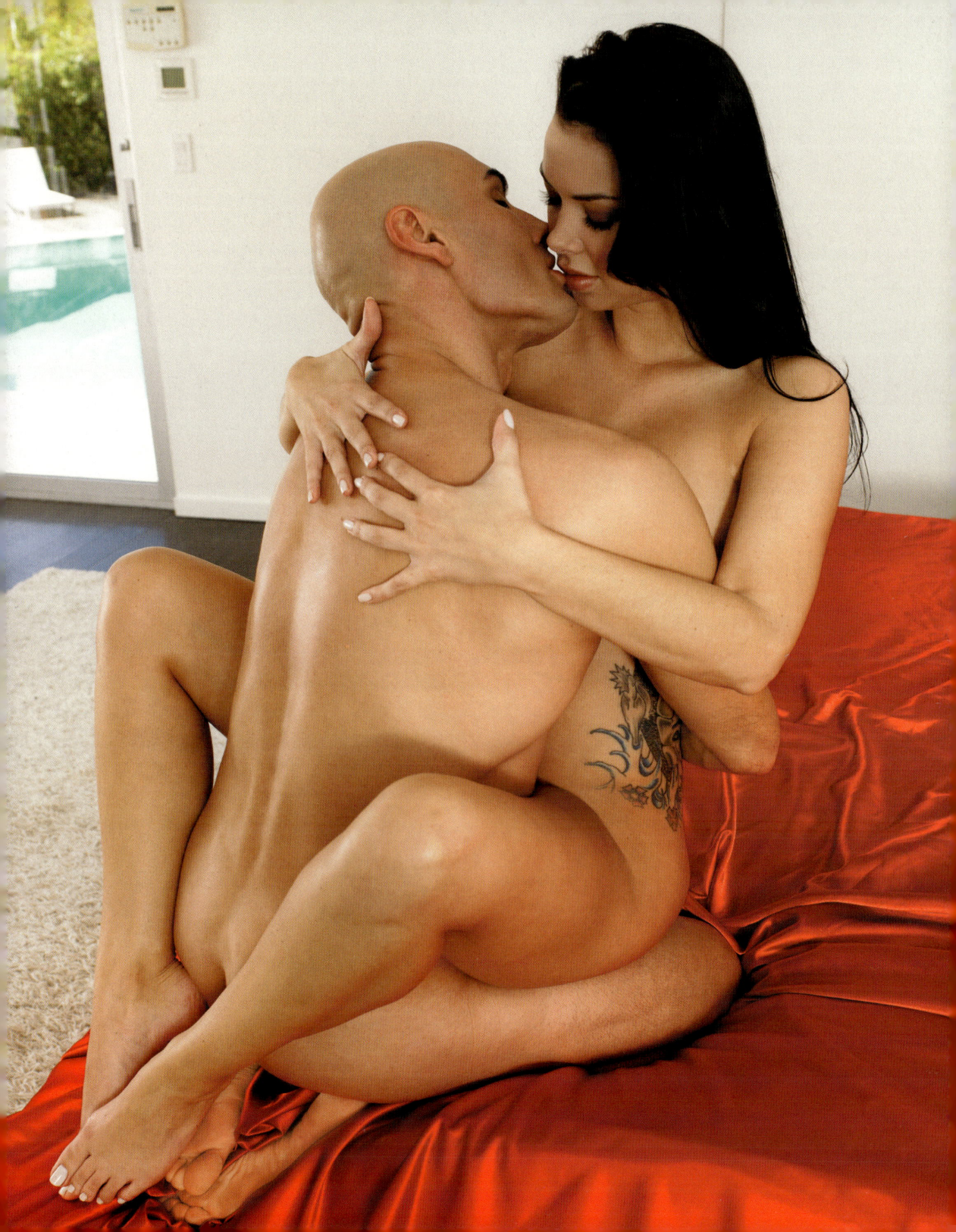

12 | ORALLY LOVING HER

{ *Worshiping the Succulent Goddess* }

VATSYAYANA DISCUSSES ORAL SEX at some length in the Kama Sutra, including the prohibitions against it from various religious teachers of the time, who said among other things that only "unchaste and wanton women" and eunuchs perform such acts. But then he sums up by saying, "In all these things connected with love, everybody should act according to the custom of his country and his own inclination."

For most women, having her yoni orally loved is one of life's most exquisite pleasures. Unlike other parts of the body that serve multiple functions, the clitoris has one sole purpose: pleasure and pleasure alone. The clitoris contains more than 8,000 nerve fibers, a higher concentration than in any other part of the human body, including the lips, fingertips, and tongue. In fact, it has twice as many as in the entire penis. Having the pearl and the entire vulva lovingly caressed with something as sensitive and moist as a mouth and tongue is profoundly erotic. It is also perhaps one of the most vulnerable and intimate of all sexual acts for women to receive.

In approaching orally loving a woman, if you come with an intention to revere and worship her most sacred place, you'll probably be a great lover. If you come with an agenda to make her climax, you may turn her off by going too fast, desensitizing her with aggressive "tongue fu" actions, or telegraphing

to her that she needs to "perform" quickly. Also, if you go down on her just to get her ready so you can penetrate her, she will likely pick up on that as well. Most women are highly intuitive, and nothing can turn them off faster than this kind of pressure.

Some women may feel self-conscious about the way that they smell, taste, or look. Men can have issues about this as well. Assuming a woman has bathed recently, a yoni simply smells and tastes, well, like a yoni. The odor and flavor vary from woman to woman, but it is usually mild. Remember that a woman's natural scent is full of pheromones specifically designed to activate the libido of her man. If either of you has concerns based on past experiences, practice "beginner's mind" and start fresh. Be present and curious, prepared to be utterly delighted by the garden of her yoni. One of the quickest ways to bring her pleasure is to find your own turn-on.

Comfort is primary for both of you. Make sure she is warm and relaxed. You can position her on the edge of the bed so you can kneel beside it or do whatever is necessary for your comfort as the "giver." Also, don't be afraid to stop in the middle if you need to. If anything, the pause will likely heighten, not diminish, her arousal. Just keep some kind of contact with her body so she doesn't feel abandoned, and tell her what you're doing. Your woman will feel it if

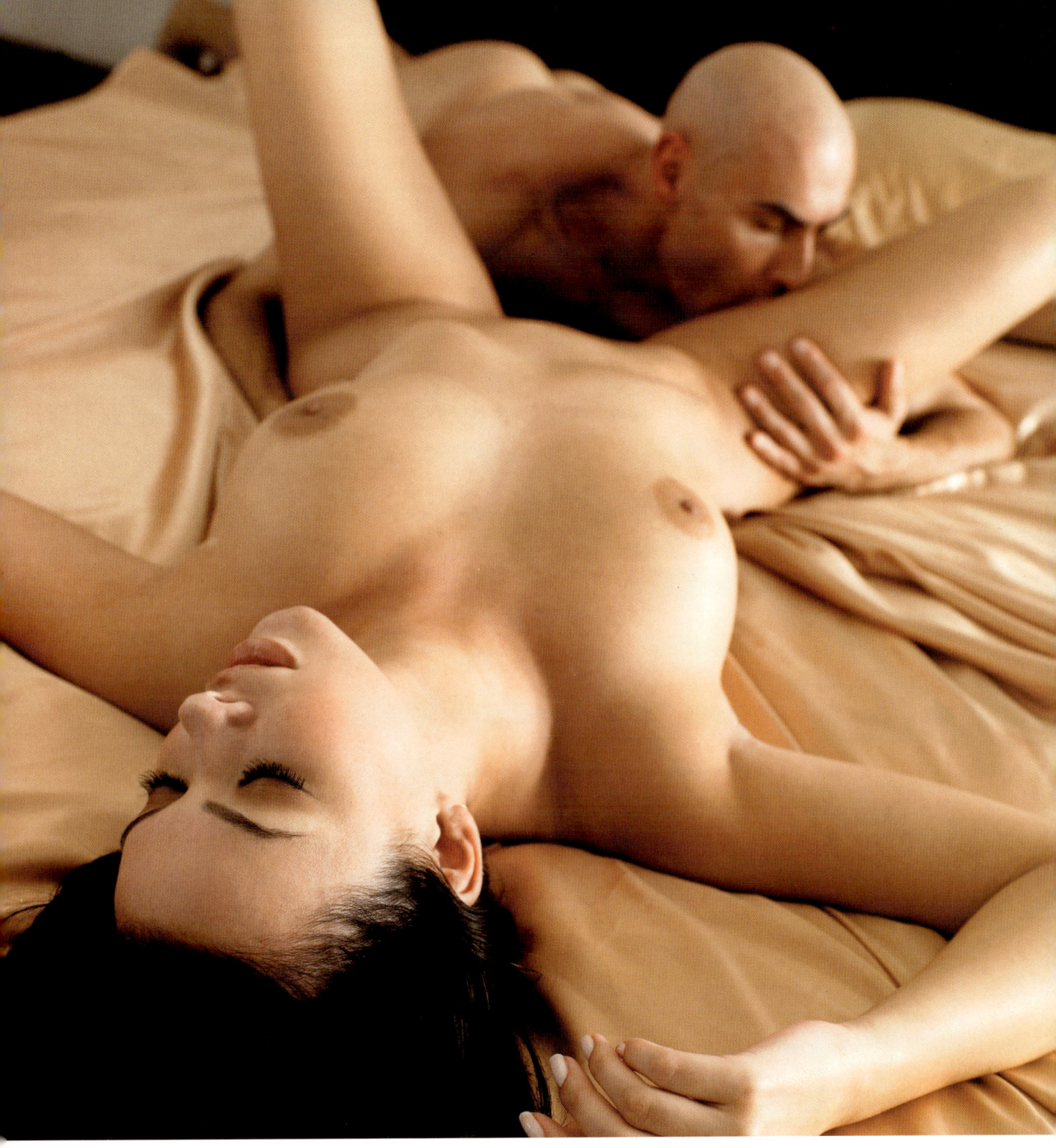

you're not "into" it, despite how well you think you're concealing it. She needs to know that you want to love her this way so that she can relax and fully receive enjoyment.

In oral loving (for her or him), keep in mind four guidelines: location, stroke, speed, and pressure. Location is critical—are you on the right spot? Stroke is the motion or movement that brings the greatest pleasure—side to side, circular, up and down, and so on. Speed covers how fast or slow you do the stroke. Pressure is about harder, firmer, softer, or gentler. Any one of these four can make or break oral sex. Good lovers give each other feedback and welcome it from their partners.

When you orally love your partner, be mindful of staying present (in the moment) with her. If you notice that you're worrying or making up stories, remind yourself to come back to the sensation of your mouth and her body. Listen to her breathing and get feedback from the sounds she's making. Or simply ask her: Does it feel good? Do you need something else? By being genuinely curious, encouraging her to share, and not taking feedback personally, you will expand your intimacy to entirely new levels.

One of the strengths of masculine energy is goal-orientation and focus. Because of this, men often appreciate it if their woman grasps their vajra quickly, right at the onset of sexual activity.

However, it can be a mistake doing this to a woman. Grabbing a woman's yoni or going down on her quickly can be startling and turn her off. Best to get her whole body involved first and *take your time*. You probably cannot go slowly enough for her. Wait until you feel her yoni begging for your touch.

Take some time to admire her yoni. Really look at it and describe the colors, textures, and shapes that you see. Share some loving words about how much you appreciate her. Now introduce your mouth. Rather than going right for the pearl, spend some time playing with her outer lips first, nibbling and nuzzling. As she heats up and opens to you, move your tongue between the outer and inner lips of her vulva as if they were a clock face, starting at the bottom (6:00) and moving up to the top (12:00) and back down again, first on one side and then on the other.

When she's well aroused, concentrate more energy on her pearl. Slide the hood back so that it is exposed, and then start by simply applying firm pressure with your whole tongue. Don't move it yet. Just stay firm and still. Let her attune to your presence without more stimulation, so that she can open more fully to you, invite you more deeply in, and meet you with her own orgasmic energy.

Then begin to flick your tongue steadily across her pearl. Try sucking it gently into your mouth and releasing it. You can also use the flat of your tongue, starting inside the well of her yoni and drawing it straight up and over her pearl. Depending on her anatomy and your own, you can also use your nose to apply pressure to the pelvic bone just above the clitoris, which is arousing for many women. Be creative with your movements—the possibilities are endless.

When you sense that she is building to climax and is wet, introduce one *well-lubricated* finger into her yoni (and later two or more) and stroke the inner walls, particularly concentrating on the front and upper part one to two inches inside, where her sacred spot is located. This will have a slightly different texture, more spongy and rougher than the smooth inner vaginal walls. After you've located the sacred spot, opposite of her clitoris, apply pressure inside as you use your tongue to apply pressure outside. Imagine a line of energy going through your mouth, meeting your finger a few inches away, and then coming back.

As she builds to orgasm, keep the movements of your mouth and fingers rhythmic. This is usually a good time to increase pressure and speed. It's also okay to take a break, slow down, or stop temporarily and allow her to integrate the surge of orgasmic energy. This is helpful if she is feeling "stuck" or pushing herself too hard toward a goal of orgasm, rather than opening more deeply, relaxing, and allowing it. Remember that when you return to

stimulation, she's already in a heightened state and going higher. (Of course, if she's very close to climaxing and you stop, that could be aggravating, but hopefully she will tell you, "Don't stop!")

As she begins to move into the orgasmic wave, continue to suck and stroke, but as she crests, begin to slow down, maintaining firm contact with her yoni. Then try applying a steady pressure but stop the movement so she feels "held" as she moves through waves of orgasmic bliss. Some women prefer only a slight easing off of stimulation and can continue to achieve additional orgasms after the first one. Stay out of your mind and in the present moment with your beloved and you cannot go wrong. Visualize sending love and pleasure into her most sacred place. Stay connected to her yoni for *as long as possible* afterward, which will give her the opportunity to integrate the orgasmic energy and become grounded.

Also, remember that a woman may be completely satisfied with your oral loving even if she does not reach orgasm. Don't feel that orgasm has to be the goal. Receiving from you in this way can be profoundly healing and pleasurable with or without orgasm.

13 | ORALLY LOVING HIM

{ Bowing Down to His Wand of Light }

MAYBE NOTHING MAKES a man feel more loved and accepted than having a woman take him inside her mouth. Like her yoni, a woman's mouth is an exquisite place of wetness, warmth, and pulsation—with the added bonus of a tongue! In the Kama Sutra, Vatsyayana speaks of a variety of ways to practice "mouth congress" on a man, including Sucking the Mango Fruit (sucking just the head) and Swallowing It Up (taking him entirely into your mouth).

Sculptures of the erect lingam are common throughout India, symbolizing the sacred masculine power of Shiva. They are always shown with a yoni at the base to affirm the interconnectedness of masculine and feminine energies in the dance of life. In addition to pleasuring your man, consider that in orally loving him you are honoring the sacred masculine inside him, with its qualities of protection, clarity, and direction. Holding the awareness of his deeper divine essence while loving your man will likely make you a great lover regardless of your technique.

Many of the tips and techniques discussed in Orally Loving Her apply to him as well. Keep in mind the four guidelines of location, stroke, speed, and pressure. Although men enjoy receiving sex orally in a variety of positions, here we invite him to lie back, relax, and practice letting go. This is also a good position for women who may have had negative experiences giving oral sex in the past because it gives her control over the depth of penetration.

Women often use their mouth like a tool, with the goal of getting him hard and getting him off as quickly as possible so that "it's over." It's much more exciting to receive oral sex when we know that our partner is getting turned on giving it to us. So when giving orally to your man, tune in to the highly sensual zones of your mouth and explore the sensations *you* feel. Explore the roof of your mouth, your lips, and under your tongue, and try sucking, licking, and flicking. Try dropping what you think you know about your partner and fellatio. Instead, investigate from a place of authentic curiosity about what turns *you* on and feels good to *both of you*.

Remember that a man doesn't have to be hard in order to feel pleasure orally, and if he's not hard, it doesn't mean that you're doing something "wrong." By loving his vajra in all its many expressions, you affirm his wholeness and stay in the present. Besides, a soft or semisoft vajra in your mouth can open up a world of oral delights for you.

For most men, watching you perform oral sex is tremendously arousing, so remind him to open his eyes, and make eye contact with him frequently. You can draw his sexual energy up his body and keep him connected to his heart by occasionally reaching out to touch his nipples, stroke his chest, or place your hand there.

Start by slowly caressing your partner's whole body. If you have long hair, drag it down his chest and across his pelvis. Take some time to admire his vajra and tell him what you appreciate about it. Men feel very honored when you tell them about the beauty and power of their vajra. Cup his deva mani (balls) and delicately rub and squeeze the skin, paying particular attention to the erotic zone of the perineum near the rear of the scrotum. You can use your mouth and very gently suck his balls into your mouth and hold them there. Moan so he can feel the vibration.

When you're ready to move to his vajra, start low on the shaft and alternate with firm squeezing of your hand and sucking or licking. Try moving around the shaft with your tongue (as if you were winding it with a ribbon). Finally, take just the tip of his vajra into your mouth and hold it there without moving for a few breaths. Then wrap your mouth around the head and flick your tongue, which will delight him. Also simply try a wide open mouth with a flat tongue and stimulate the highly sensitive underside of his shaft where the frenulum is located (the triangular area just below the tip and hole on the underside of the vajra).

You can also hold him firmly at the base of his vajra with one hand while you use the thumb and forefinger of your other hand to circle him just under the tip. Then you can move the circles up and down in a twisting motion while you pleasure the head continually with your tongue. As with the clitoris on a woman, be creative with your movements—the possibilities are endless.

As he builds toward orgasm, he will likely want you to increase the pressure as well as your speed, simulating intercourse. Remember to keep things very moist with lots of saliva, particularly if you are doing a lot of manual stimulation. The wetter it is, the better it will feel to him. By continuing to hold him firmly around the base, you can prevent him from penetrating you more deeply than you would like. As he nears climax, you can bring him to a new level of ecstasy by applying gentle pressure with your thumb or forefinger (watch your nails) to his perineum (the spot between his scrotum and anus).

If you're uncomfortable swallowing, make sure that you discuss this with your partner beforehand so he can tell you when he's about to ejaculate. However, swallowing is not so difficult, the taste is mild, semen is loaded with energy, and your man will love you for it. Even better, relax and continue to hold him in your mouth after he ejaculates until his erection subsides. Allow him the ecstatic feeling of nesting inside your mouth as he basks in the afterglow of his orgasm. Most men have never had their vajra loved this way, and it can be a profoundly moving experience for them.

14 | SACRED CIRCLE

{ *Sixty-Nine Is Divine* }

ALTHOUGH WE COMMONLY REFER to simultaneous oral sex with a partner as "69," the Kama Sutra says, "When a man and woman lie down in an inverted order, with the head of one towards the feet of the other and carry on this congress, it is called 'Congress of a Crow.'" (I guess the crows in ancient India were more creative than those squawking in my backyard—although this position would certainly keep them quiet.) I like the name Sacred Circle because when you engage in orally loving each other this way, a golden circuit of energy is created between you that can bring you to a new level of oneness.

The challenge some people have with the position is the feeling of having a split focus: When you're enjoying the receiving, you may forget about giving, and vice versa. With some practice and a focus on the idea of one circuit of energy looping between you, the polarity of giving and receiving blurs, and you'll increasingly find yourself unable to distinguish between the sensations you feel in your mouth as you pleasure your beloved and the pleasure you feel in your genitals as you receive his or her loving. You may even come to experience the feeling that you are simultaneously playing the music and being the instrument at the same time. This is the oneness of the Sacred Circle.

Although this position is also delightful and very sexy with one partner on top of the other, here we'll focus on the side-by-side version to "equalize" you and emphasize your unity.

To begin, put your attention on the flow of sexual energy between you rather than focusing on performing or bringing your partner to orgasm. With his mouth on her yoni and her mouth on his vajra, you are in an ideal, energetic loop. To create the circle of orgasmic energy, the man visualizes breathing love, pleasure, and devotion out of his mouth and into the yoni of his beloved. He sees it flowing into her hips, where it moves up her body, through her heart, and into her mouth. In her mouth it is magnified and breathed back into his vajra. Through his vajra it travels up his body and back into his mouth where he, once again, breathes it back into her. And the circle continues with the woman visualizing herself giving energy through her mouth into his sex chakra, and seeing it travel in a sacred loop up his body, out of his mouth, into her yoni, and up her body to her mouth again.

Use your inhalations and exhalations to build this golden circle of orgasmic energy between you. Listen to your partner and find the rhythm together. After a while, you can agree to reverse the direction of the circle. A little tricky! Now instead of your

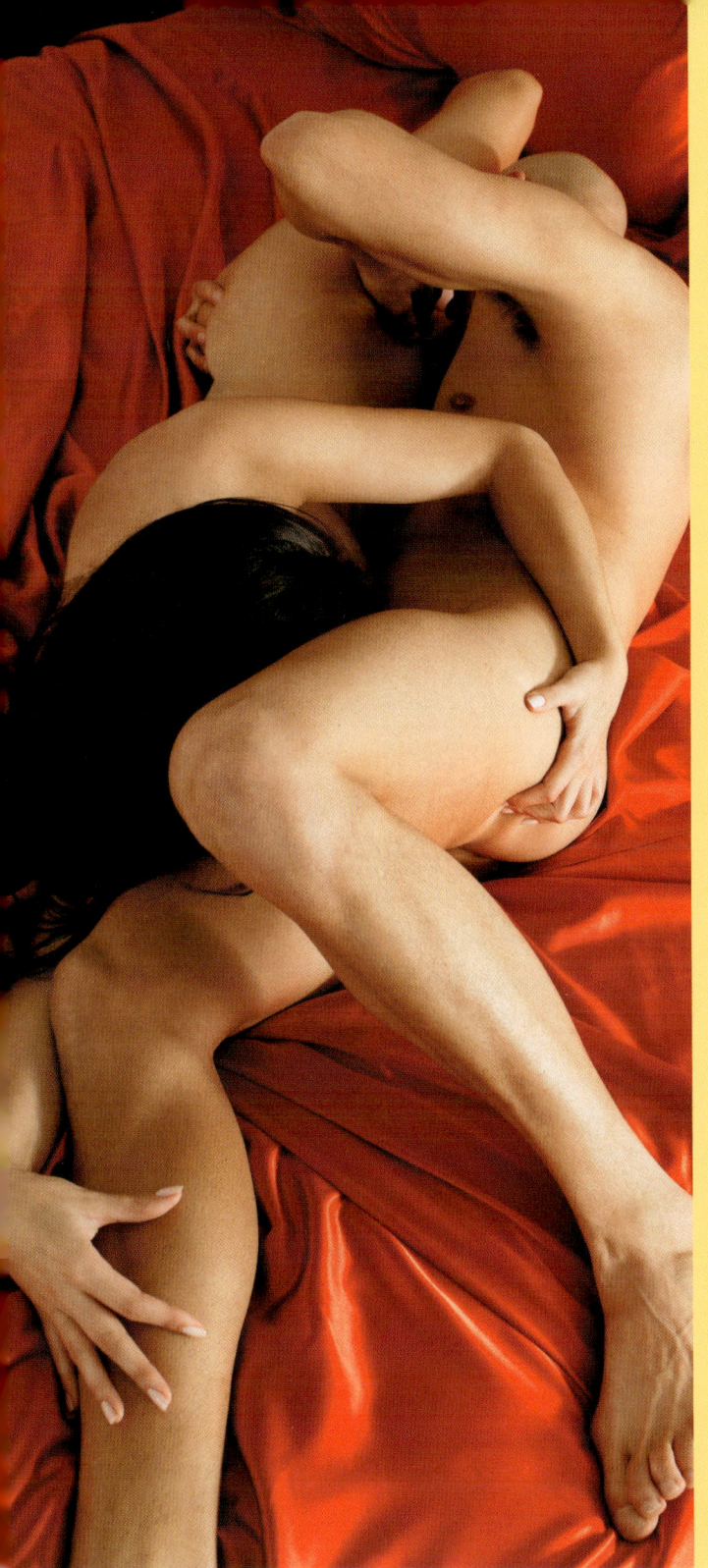

mouth giving energy *to* your beloved, imagine that it is receiving energy *from* his or her genitals. See it moving into your mouth and down your body and into your sex chakra, where you then give it back to your partner's mouth and it travels down his or her body the same way. Notice the differences in how the energy feels moving up the spine versus moving down. Moving up will bring you more in contact with the spiritual and heavenly realms. Moving the energy down is grounding and will connect you more solidly to the earthly realm.

It can be a lovely moment of grace to experience a simultaneous climax, but don't pressure yourselves by making that a goal. Although they seem to do it effortlessly in movies, it's fairly uncommon between real lovers. However, in this posture with the breathing exercise, the extreme interconnectedness, and the very direct oral stimulation, it's one of the better positions to give you a shot at coming together. Just don't work too hard at it. If one or both of you move toward orgasm in the Sacred Circle, do remember to stay mindful of your teeth in the height of your passion.

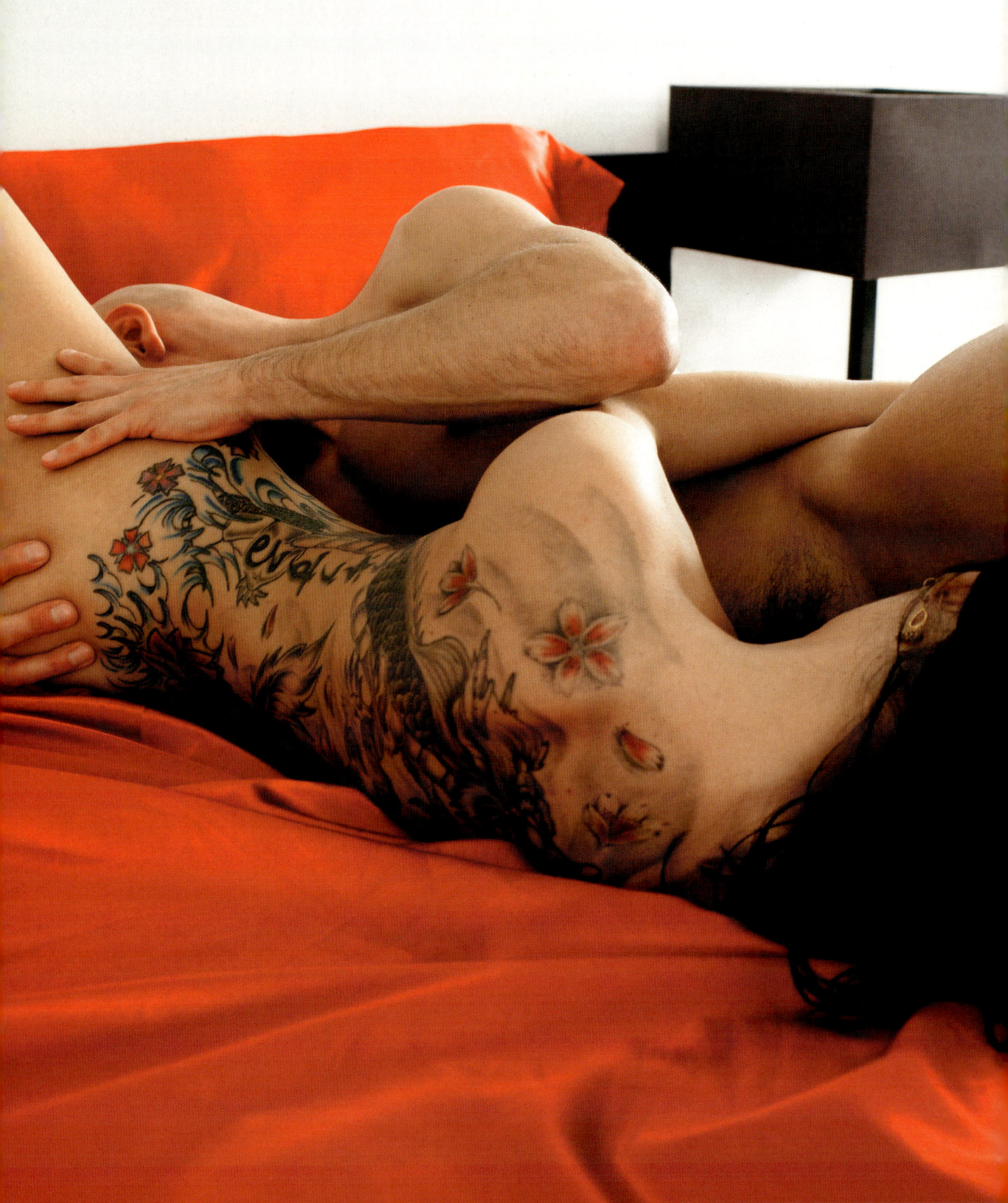

Making Time for Sex

If you've just fallen in love, sex is at the top of your priority list. Why go to the movies or out to dinner if you can cozy up by the fireplace and make love? If you're in a longer-term relationship, sex can be relegated to the very end of the day when you're exhausted or squeezed into the morning before you rush off into busyness (although those quickie sex sessions can be delicious!). Modern life is full of demands on our time, and the reality is, we always make time for what's most important to us. So if lovemaking isn't happening as often or for as long as you'd like, it's time for some reevaluation.

Schedule a full or half day with nothing to do but make love, and calendar it regularly. That doesn't have to mean having intercourse the whole time. Explore one another's bodies, touch, lick, suck, share what you appreciate about each other, bathe together, soul gaze, read love poems to one another, nap, cuddle, be creative. Think of making love this way: there is more love present than when you began. Another way to think of it: making love present.

If you're a parent busy running around all the time handling your child's activities, here's a reminder: there's *nothing* more important to your children than their parents being *together* and being *happy*—so invest time in your relationship.

Create an Altar

Another way to invoke the sacred in your lovemaking is to create an altar. It can be as simple or elaborate as you'd like. You can even transform a hotel room into a sacred space by packing a few items and creating an altar when traveling.

Find a small table, cover it with a cloth, and decorate it with items that remind you of sensuality and love: photos of you and your lover, shells from your tropical vacation, cards or small gifts you've given to each other. Make sure that the masculine and feminine are both represented— perhaps an erect crystal or statue along with rounded stones or flower petals. When you're out together, keep your eyes open for items that you both love. You can also include symbols from your own spiritual or religious tradition. The altar can be simply a part of your sacred space or you can use it to sit in front of while soul gazing, meditating, or performing a ritual together.

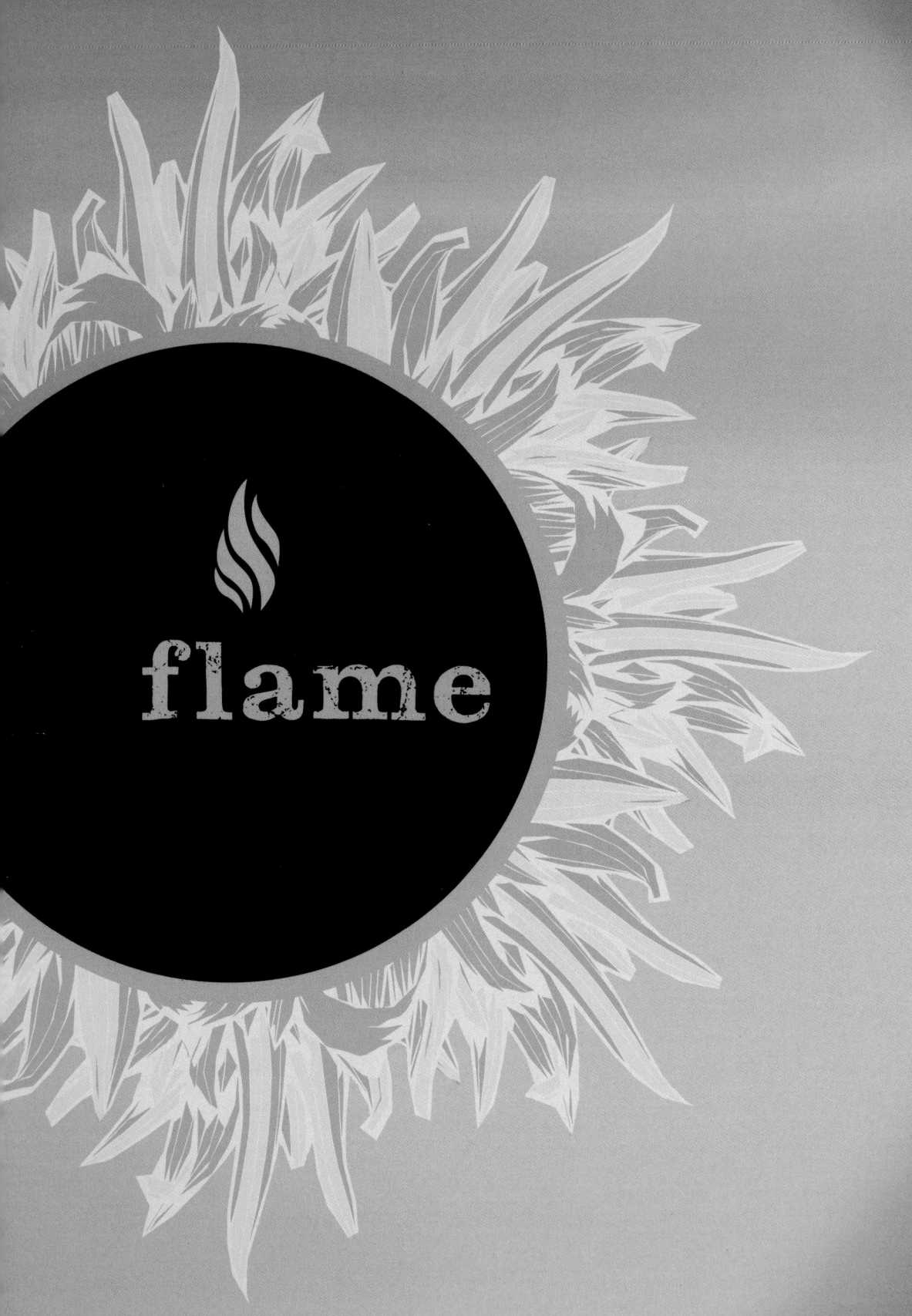

flame

THE SPARK OF THE MATCH
FLARES BRIGHTLY INTO A
FLAME. WE WATCH THE GOLDEN
LIGHT GATHER STRENGTH. A
BLENDED SPECTRUM—WHITE,
GOLD, ORANGE, RED, AND BLUE—
THE DISTANCE DISSOLVING
BETWEEN ME AND YOU. FANNING
THE FLAMES OF DESIRE, YOUR
KAMA SUTRA PATH MOVES INTO
WARMER TERRITORY WITH
POSTURES THAT WILL FLUSH
YOUR CHEEKS AND QUICKEN
YOUR PULSE.

15 | YAB YUM

{ The Yummiest of Unions }

ONE OF THE MOST BEAUTIFUL Kama Sutra postures, Yab Yum represents the unity of Shiva and Shakti, or masculine and feminine, in ultimate oneness. In the East, deities are commonly shown enthroned on the sacred lotus flower. In this position, the man's lap becomes the royal seat for his goddess. A perfect posture for warming up and building energy, it allows you to embrace, gaze deeply at each other, and kiss passionately. And when you add breath and movement to that kindling, watch out—things will heat up quickly!

① The man sits cross-legged with a few strategically placed pillows: one under his butt so his hips tilt forward and are higher than his knees, and one under each knee (if needed) so that he can relax and be supported. His back is straight with his hands resting on his knees.

② The woman then lowers herself onto his lap and, if possible, wraps her legs around his waist with the soles of her feet touching behind him. She may also place a pillow under her butt for support. At this point, all the energy centers are aligned between partners, including the genitals, heart, and head. Prior to intercourse, the man's vajra should be positioned up and the woman's yoni lips can be pressed against or wrapped around it in an embrace. Here you can soul gaze while breathing deeply in unison, drawing the sexual energy up the spine and exhaling it into your partner.

③ Finally, when the man is erect and the woman is hungry for penetration, she can rise up slightly and lower herself onto his vajra. On her inhalation, she drops her head back, arches slightly, and tilts her pelvis back.

④ On her exhalation, she tilts her head and pelvis forward, drawing her abdomen in toward her spine. Her man mirrors her movements and breathes the same way. The rocking motion along with the breathing will activate the kundalini, or sexual energy that resides at the base of the spine.

⑤ Once you have mastered moving in unison, try alternating movements (the woman inhaling and arching as the man exhales and concaves). This will create a rocking rhythm with different sensations and pleasures.

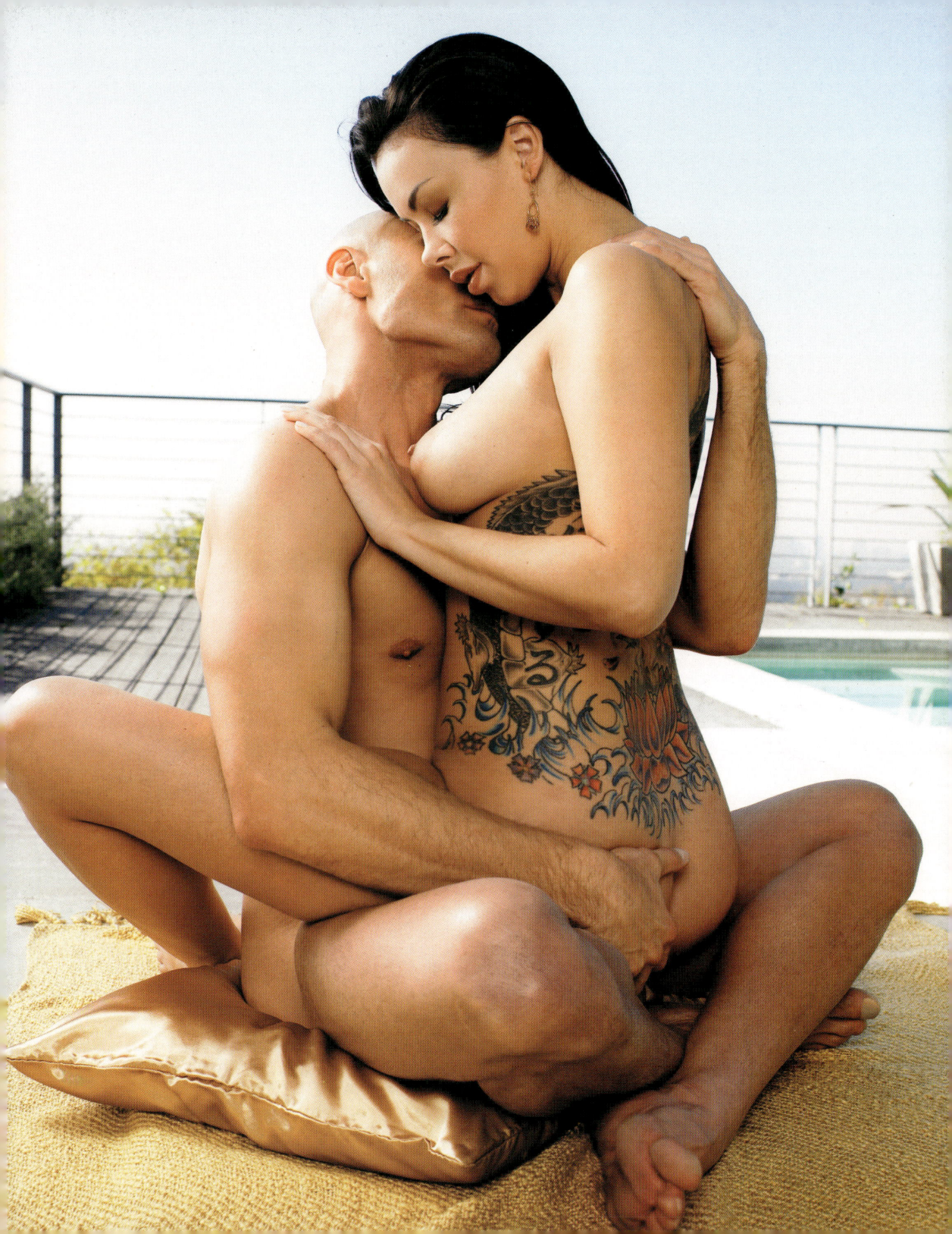

16 | ROLLING POSTURE

{ A Variation of Yab Yum }

IN THIS VARIATION OF YAB YUM, gentle movements by both the man and the woman allow lovers to explore more subtle sensations in sexual union. Good for balancing masculine and feminine energy, the posture calls for mutual participation and harmony in your movements. By facing each other, you can look deep into your partner's eyes and soul gaze, softening the focus on the surface personality and allowing yourself to be drawn into the deeper divinity within.

① The man sits upright, either cross-legged or with the soles of his feet together, creating a "seat" for the woman. He should place a firm pillow or folded blanket under his butt so that his hips are slightly elevated and place pillows under his legs (if needed) to support his knees.

② The woman sits between his legs, wrapping her legs around him so that her feet touch, or placing her feet together on the floor behind him. Here you can soul gaze, kiss, and embrace one another as you build sexual energy.

③ Next, the woman holds the man's neck or shoulder with one hand and uses her other hand to raise the opposite leg up slightly, lifting that foot off the floor. By alternating sides, she can explore the variety of feelings in different areas of her yoni; she can also use the leg movement to shorten or tighten her yoni.

④ At the same time, the man rolls his hips from side to side to vary the sensations you both experience. He can either hold on to her hip or butt opposite of the leg that she is lifting or place both hands on the floor behind him with straight arms to support himself.

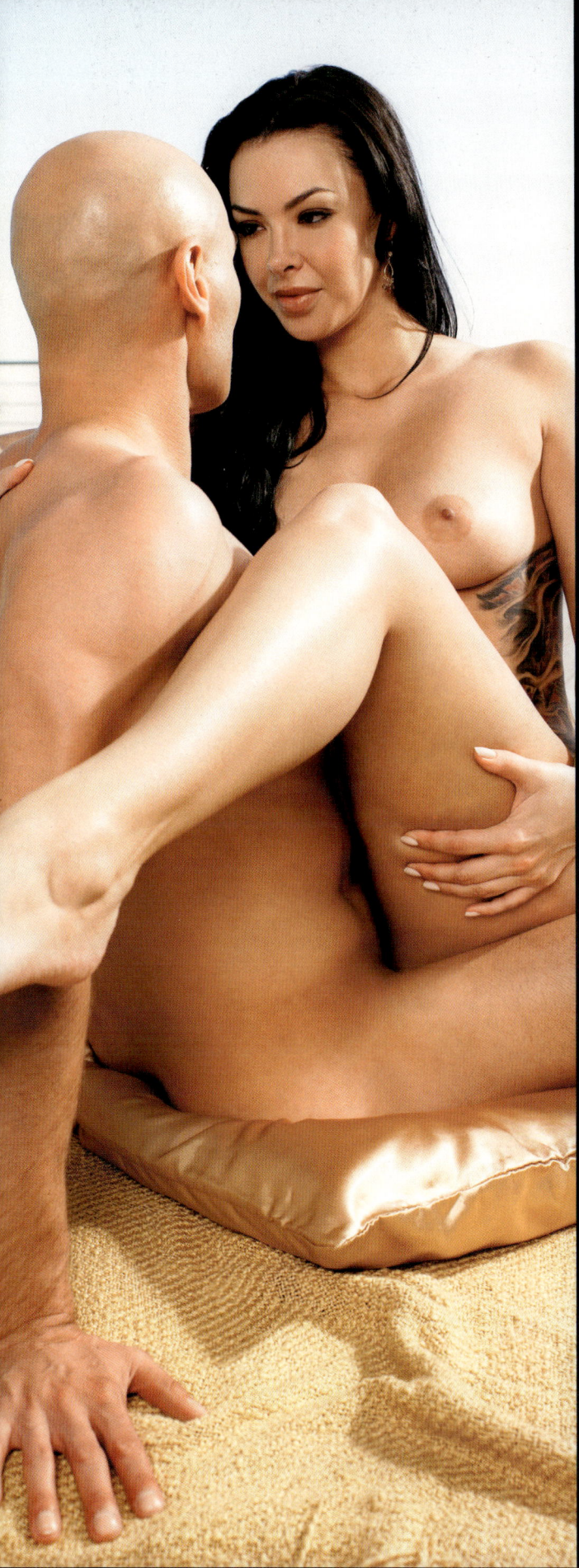

The Love Pump

This simple exercise has perhaps more power than any other to awaken sexual energy and transform your lovemaking. Commonly known as a Kegel exercise, after the gynecologist who popularized it, I like to refer to it as the Love Pump. The exercise involves contracting your pubococcygeus, or PC, muscle. This is the muscle that you use to stop the flow of urine midstream—both men and women have it.

The health benefits of having a strong PC muscle are substantial, which is why Kegel exercises are so frequently recommend by doctors. What you may not know is how great having a strong PC muscle can be for your sex life. Do your Love Pump exercises daily by rhythmically contracting and releasing the muscle. See if you can work up to 100 Love Pumps per day. You can do them anytime, anywhere, and no one will know. It's a muscle that gets in shape very fast and will soon bring you an abundance of pleasure.

For women, using the Love Pump on your partner's vajra while he's inside you can eventually be even more orgasmic for him than thrusting. And, as you strengthen your PC and vaginal muscles, you bring vitality and healing blood flow to your yoni, increasing your own sexual desire and responsiveness. It's even possible to eventually bring yourself to orgasm just by doing the Love Pump. Hands-free orgasms, ladies—imagine the possibilities!

For men, a strong Love Pump can give you greater ejaculatory control. You'll be able to last longer and eventually may even be able to have multiple orgasms without ejaculating if you practice. This could be the most golden of all the sacred sexuality tips, because this simple exercise can radically transform your responsiveness and increase your sexual pleasure. So do your Love Pumps every day!

17 | JEWEL CASE

{ A Rear-Entry Gem }

THIS REAR-ENTRY POSTURE has the benefit of creating a snug fit for the man's vajra while also allowing him to relax with his back supported as he enjoys the view of his woman from behind, riding his erection. For the woman, it allows for easy access to clitoral stimulation, plus the angle of penetration can allow her to explore and awaken new pleasure spots inside her yoni.

① The man sits with his legs outstretched, knees open, to accommodate the size of his woman's hips. He leans against a piece of furniture or even a wall cushioned by a pillow. The woman nestles between his legs with her back to him. While building arousal, the man can place his vajra "up" between the cleft of her butt while kissing the back of her neck and caressing her. He can invite her to relax completely against him and surrender to his masculine strength and embrace. This is a very heart-opening posture for a woman, engendering love and trust.

② The woman can seductively press her butt against him, rotating slowly and arching her pelvis forward and back while stroking his thighs. When he is erect and she is ready, she lifts herself up and lowers herself down on his vajra. Either or both lovers can provide the movement for stimulation. Not a position for deep thrusting, this posture encourages awareness of more subtle feelings, which can build orgasmic energy.

③ The woman can place her hands on the outside of his thighs, and with straight arms support the weight of her upper body as she rocks or rotates on his erection. The man can support his weight by placing his hands on either side of his hips and straightening his arms. He can use his arms and upper body strength to tilt his pelvis toward her and move inside her. Or you can alternate who moves, with one person relaxing in the receiving while the other provides the action, building delicious passion together.

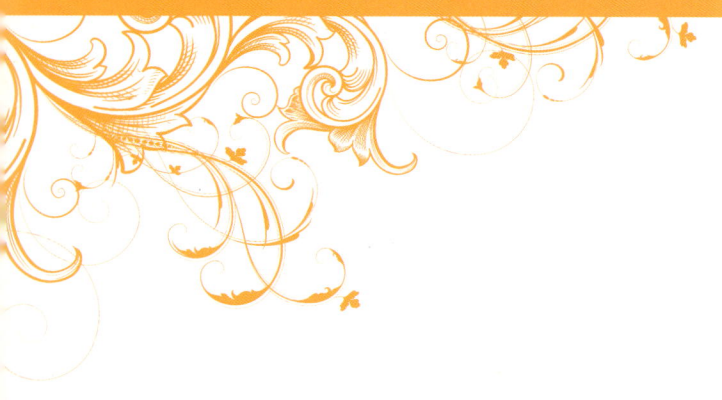

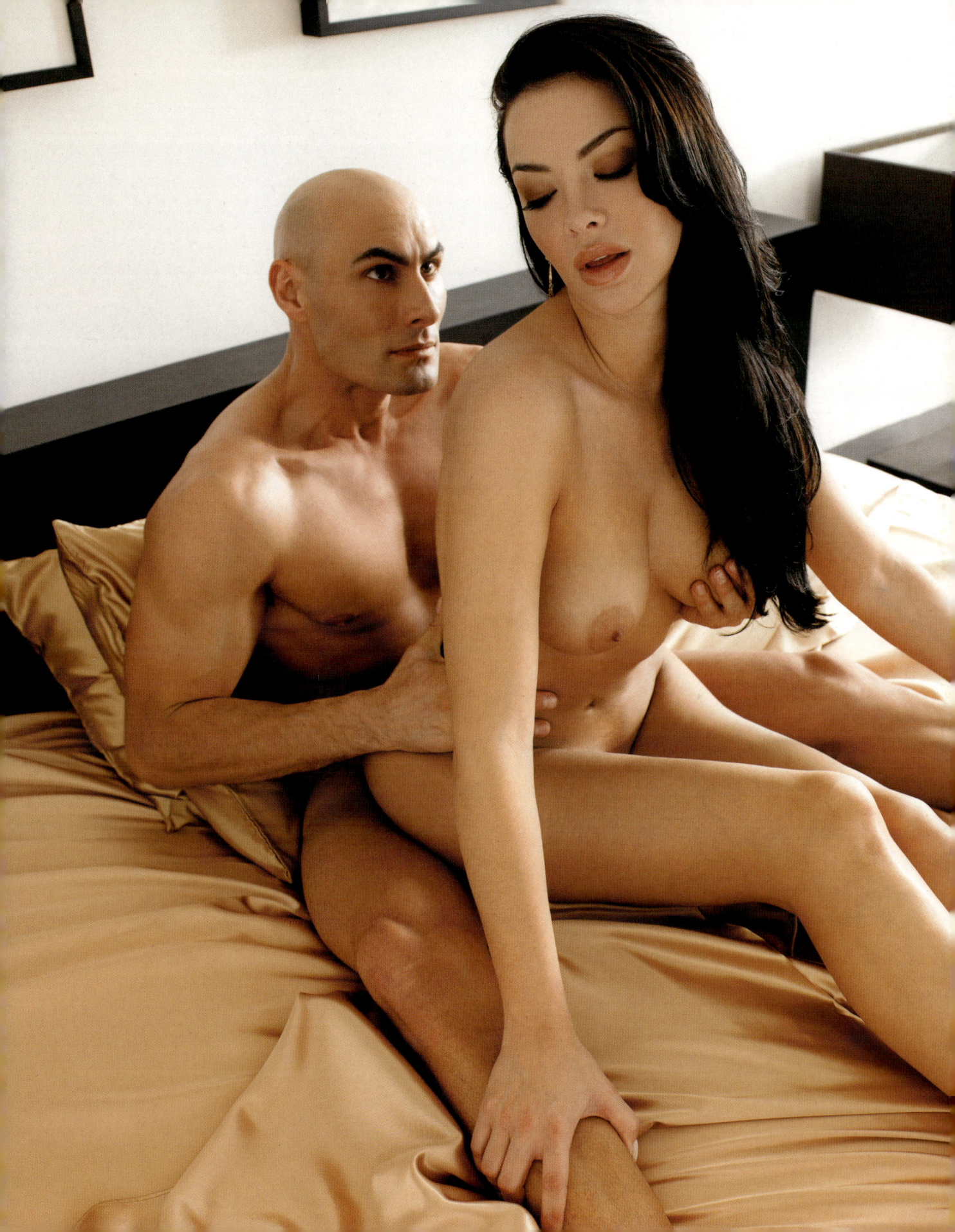

18 | SWALLOW

{ Deep Fulfillment of Desire }

ALTHOUGH THE KAMA SUTRA makes ample use of animal names, this position is not likely named after the small bird but rather the depth with which the woman can "swallow" up her lover with her yoni. The tighter fit and deeper penetration in this position can be highly pleasurable for both men and women.

"The true liberation of eroticism lies in accepting the fact that there are a million facets to it. We have, first of all, to dispense with guilt concerning its expansion, then remain open to its surprises, varied expressions, and (to add my personal formula for the full enjoyment of it) fuse it with individual love and passion for a particular human being, mingle it with dreams, fantasies, and emotion for it to attain its highest potency."

— *Anaïs Nin,* In Favor of the Sensitive Man

① The woman lies on her back, bringing her knees together and into her chest. This fully exposes her yoni to her lover and also alters the shape of it, making it tighter and shorter. The man will likely find this pose very visually stimulating. He can tease her by gently using just the tip of his vajra on her yoni to heighten the sexual energy between them.

② Once he enters her, she places her ankles around his neck, resting them on his shoulders. Depending on her flexibility, she may even fold herself in half so that her thighs press against her breasts. He leans forward as well and can even passionately kiss her if she is limber enough. She can hold on to her man's arms, gripping his biceps.

③ Alternatively, she can throw her arms above her head in a gesture of deep surrender. This will also open her heart and throat chakras to promote deeper feeling and expression. The man can then intertwine his fingers with hers and "pin" her with his love and desire.

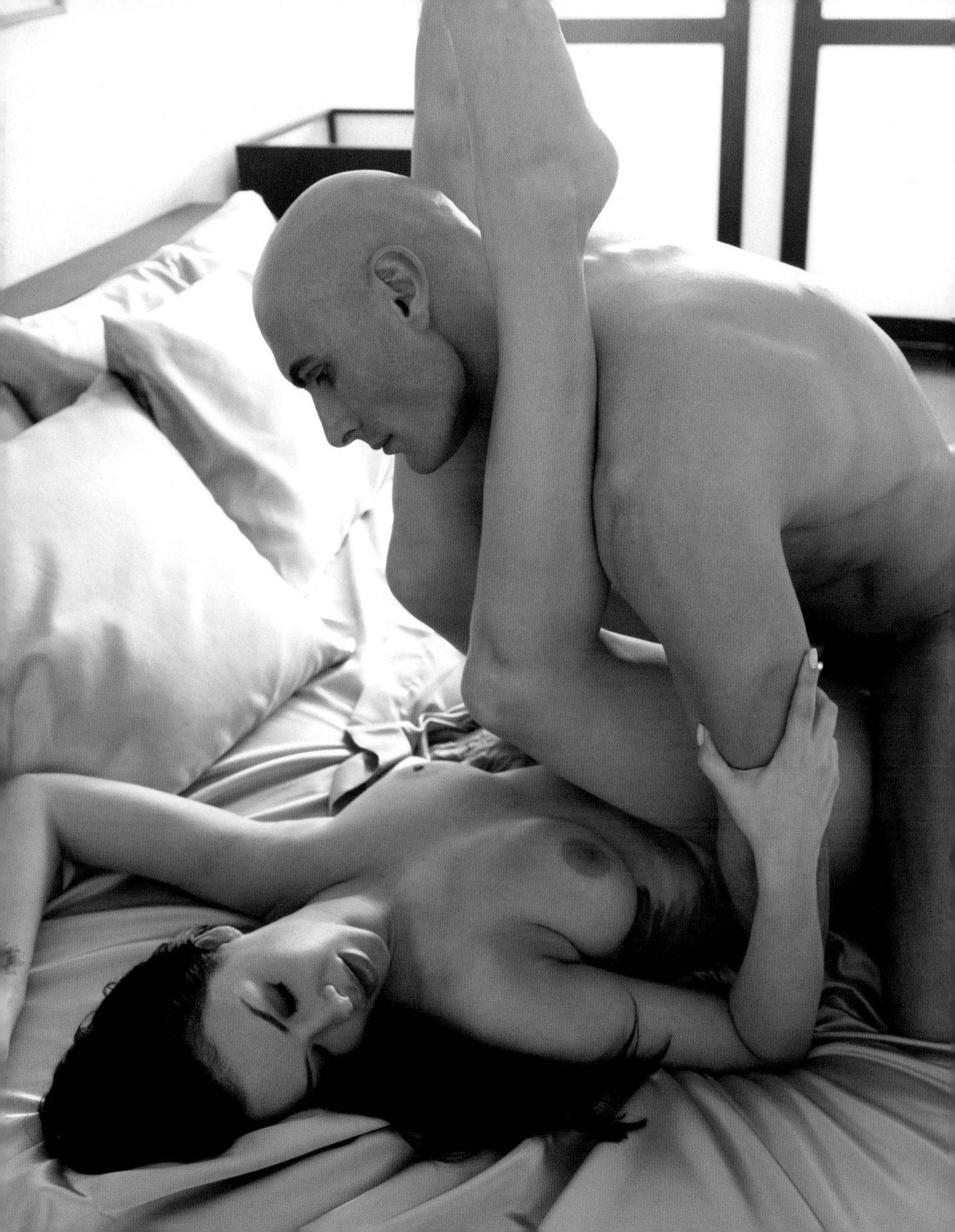

19 | PRESSED POSITION

{ A Push and Pull of Pleasure }

THIS ALTERNATIVE POSITION to Swallow, simply and aptly called Pressed Position by Vatsyayana, gives you the same benefits but with some variations to awaken new delicious sensations. Because the man is more upright, he can enjoy a better view of the action. With her feet placed flat on his chest rather than on his shoulders, the woman can more actively participate in their erotic dance. Activating her feet will also help "ground" her if she's feeling spacey or living too much in her head.

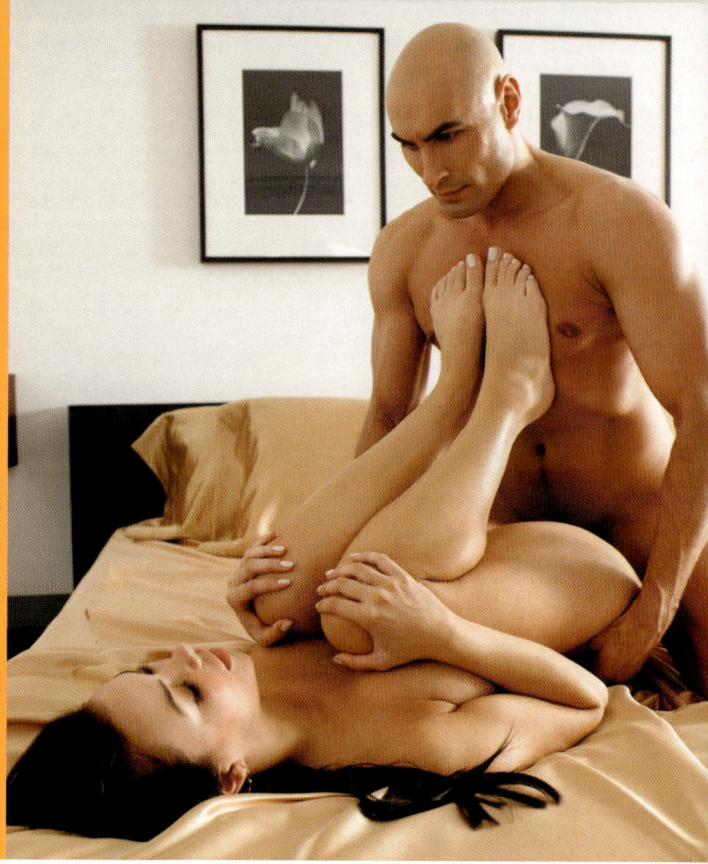

① The woman lies on her back with her knees bent and together, placing the soles of her feet flat against the man's chest. She keeps her legs pressed together during the position and holds on to her knees.

② The man kneels in front of her, bringing his hips and pelvis in alignment with her yoni in order to enter her. He can lift her hips up with his hands or place pillows underneath her to raise her to the right height. His knees are open wide and placed on either side of her hips. He holds on to her hips to control the movement and depth of his thrusting, remembering to alternate between shallow and deeper penetration. He can build sexual energy by teasing her with the tip of his vajra until she is begging him to take her fully.

③ In this posture, the woman can use her feet against his chest to meet his thrusting with movements of her own, or raise her hips and adjust the angle of her pelvis (tilting forward or back, to one side or the other) to target sensation where it feels most pleasurable to her. As he penetrates her, she can feel the beating of his heart and the power of his chest as it rocks against and sends energy into the soles of her feet.

④ The man can also alternate between active and receptive roles. If she is more active, then he can relax back by placing his hands behind him with straight arms for support while pressing his pelvis forward and enjoying the sensation of his beloved gyrating and rocking her pelvis on his vajra.

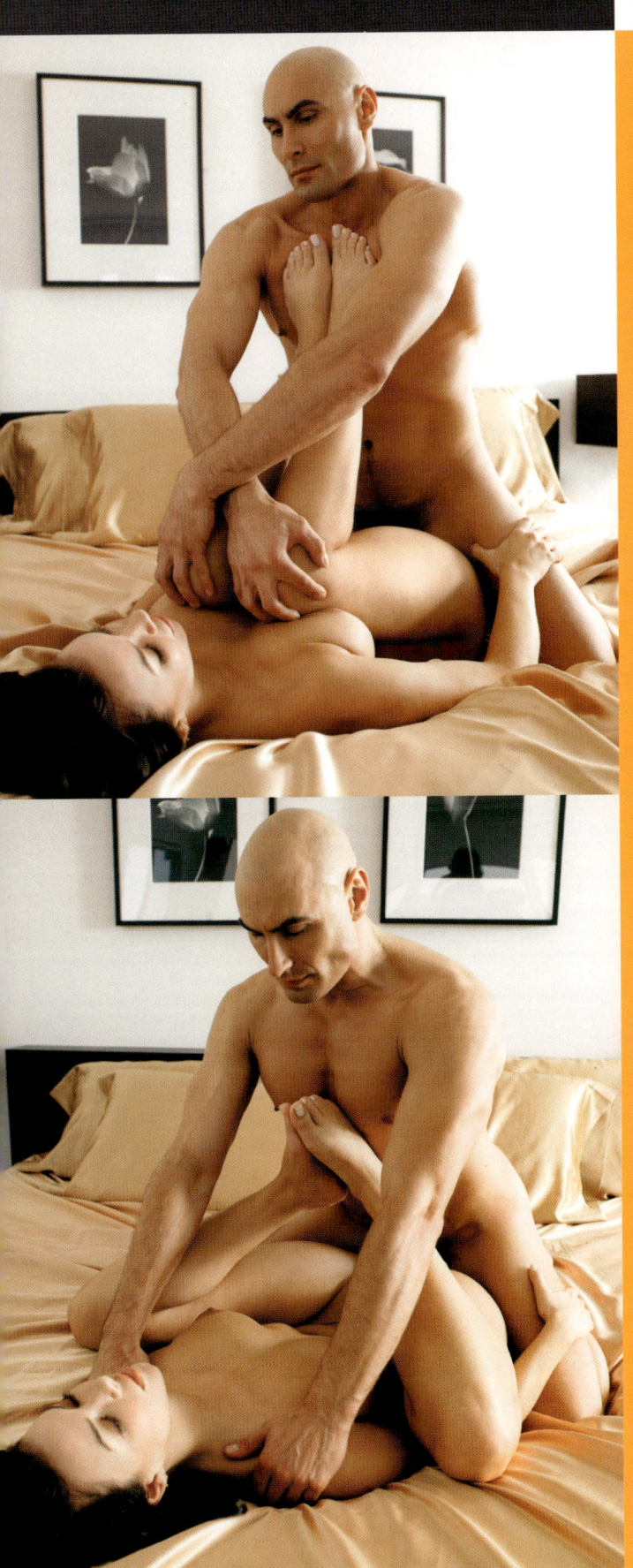

PUJA

20

{ A Variation of the Pressed Position }

AS AN ALTERNATIVE ARM POSITION for the man, he crosses his hands at the wrist, his right hand holding her right knee, left hand holding her left knee. A puja is a Sanskrit term for a form of worship or a sacred circle. By crossing his hands at the wrist, the man's arms create a circle of heart energy he can send to his beloved. He will also have more strength in this position to press her knees together so she can relax her legs while her yoni hugs his vajra more tightly.

THE CRAB

21

{ A Sideways Variation of the Pressed Position }

IN A THIRD ALTERATIVE, the woman places her feet on her man's chest but with the soles of her feet together and her knees splaying open. Rather than the man thrusting forward and back, the woman engages in a side-to-side motion, the way a crab scuttles. For many women, side-to-side movements can be tremendously healing and very pleasurable. The man remains motionless and offers his vajra as a healing tool for his woman to use as she explores the movements that bring her the most pleasure (which will most certainly bring him pleasure as well).

22 | ROSE IN BLOOM

{ *Watch Her Blossom* }

THIS CAN BE A DEEPLY RELAXING and sensual posture for both lovers. By leaning against a piece of furniture, the man's back is supported, leaving his hands free to caress his beloved or rock her against him. The woman lies on her back with her legs elevated, concentrating the flow of sexual energy into her pelvis.

① The man sits in front of a couch, chair, or low bed with his legs outstretched in front of him and his back well supported. The woman lies down between his legs, her feet pointing toward him, stretching out long and breathing deeply so that her chest expands, like a rose in bloom. This is a perfect opportunity for the man to take a few moments to gaze at his partner in admiration and share some words of appreciation with her as she practices receiving his love and enjoys being "seen."

② When you are both ready, the man can gently reach out and pull his partner to him by her hips or she can seductively inch herself forward so that he may enter her.

③ She raises her legs up to rest on his shoulders while he begins rocking his pelvis and finding a rhythm that pleases them both. He can try rotating his hips clockwise and then counterclockwise for different sensations. This is also an ideal position for stimulating the woman's clitoris, something the man can do for her or she can do for herself, allowing him to watch her growing pleasure.

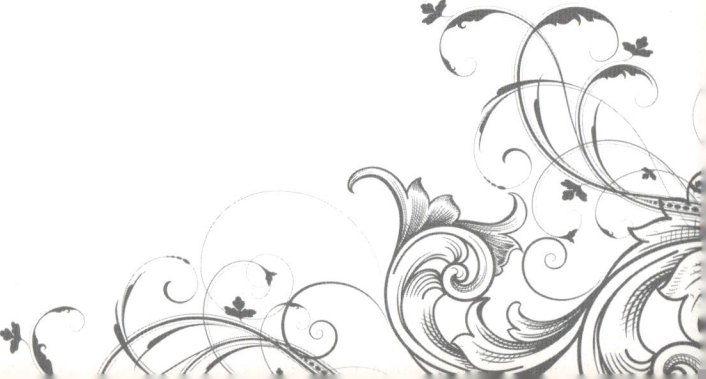

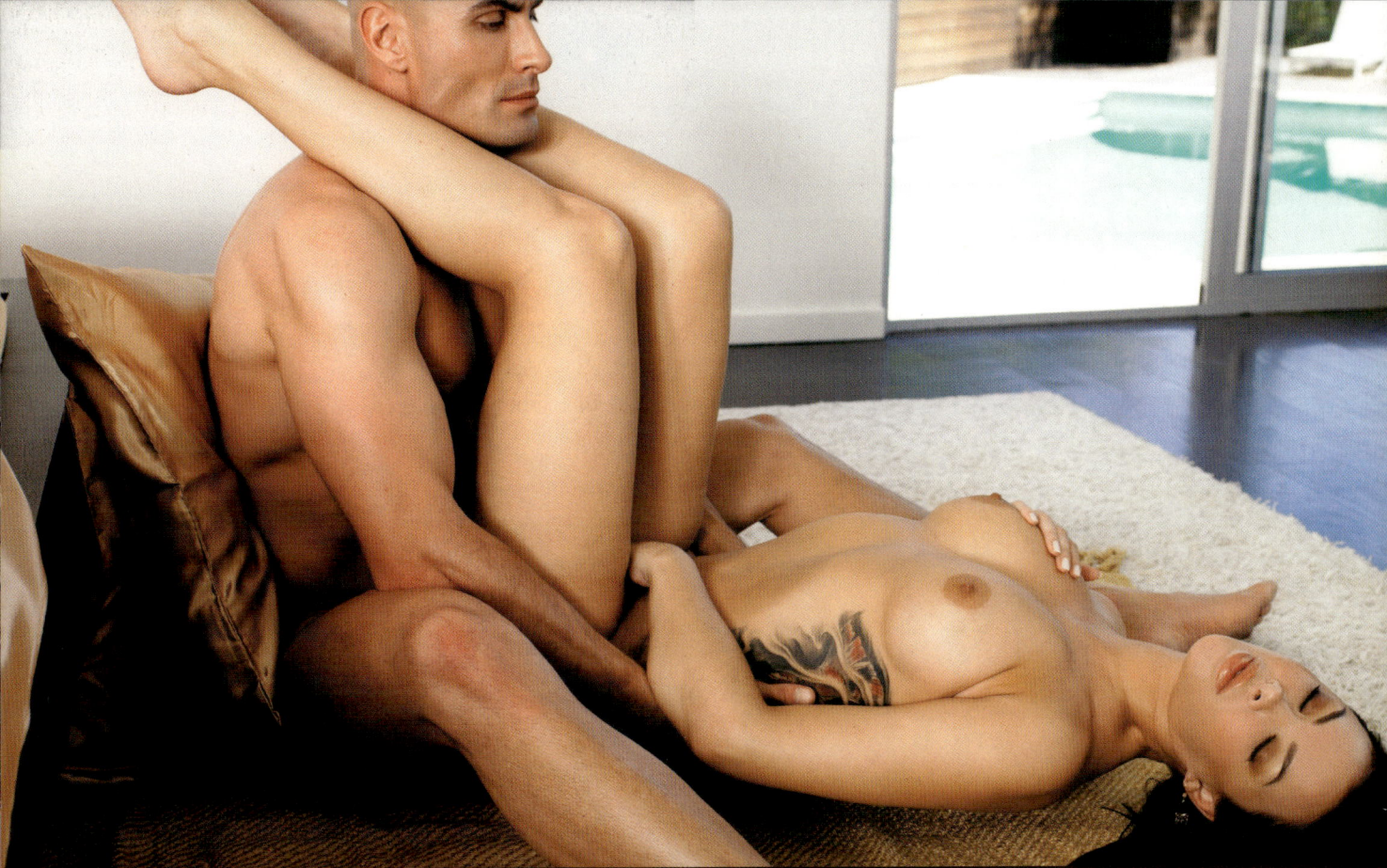

Breath of Life

Because breathing seems so basic, it's easy to dismiss. But if you want to be the ultimate Kama Sutra lover and take your sexuality beyond where it's ever been, breathing is your ticket. First of all, most people breathe at only a fraction of their capacity. Increasing the amount of oxygen you take in calms the mind, enlivens the body, brings you into the present moment, positively affects brain chemistry by boosting dopamine (the "feel good" neurochemical)—the list goes on and on. When you breathe in rhythm with your partner, you increase arousal levels, supercharge sensation everywhere, and intensify orgasms.

There are many different ways to breathe together. Practice by slowing down and deepening the breath, inhaling and exhaling to a count of six or more. You can do this in unison or alternate (you

breathe in while your partner breathes out). To pump up the sexual energy, try the Fire Breath. Keep your mouth closed and exhale through your nose with short, rapid bursts, pulling your stomach muscles in to pump the air out. Don't worry about the inhalation—it happens automatically. Do this for three minutes, then rest with normal breathing and repeat if desired. Also pay attention to your breathing as you move into orgasm. Women in particular have a tendency to barely breathe or worse, hold their breath. You will take your orgasms to entirely new levels if you use your breath. As you inhale, imagine "sucking" the orgasmic energy from your pelvis up your spine to the crown of your head. Using your breathing in this way is key to experiencing whole-body orgasms. As things heat up between you and your lover, keep coming back to the breath.

23 | CAMEL'S HUMP

{ A Standing Rear-Entry Position }

THIS REAR-ENTRY POSITION is ideal for deep penetration. Men will enjoy it because they can stand comfortably while admiring how sexy their partner is from behind. Depending on the flexibility of the woman, she can relax her spine, let go of tension in her shoulders, and enjoy being deeply filled. The inversion will also bring fresh blood and energy to her head.

Get Slippery

The importance of lubrication cannot be overemphasized. The wetter it is, the better it's going to feel for both of you. A woman's natural lubrication varies a great deal depending on her cycle, hormones, mood, age, and other factors. It is not necessarily an indication of how turned on she is—she can be very excited and not wet, or vice versa. Best to ask.

Find a lubricant that you both like (preferably as natural as possible because the woman will "ingest" it immediately into her system through her yoni) and always have it on hand. Use it liberally and be playful about it so the woman doesn't feel judged or embarrassed. Also, because the vaginal tissue can be so sensitive, always lick or lubricate your fingers before touching her yoni. She will open and receive you much more readily that way.

① The woman bends forward, facing away from her man, and curves her spine up like a camel's hump. If she's flexible enough, she can place her hands on the floor. If not, she can place them on her calves anywhere below her knees, or she can use cushions or bolsters in front of her for comfort and stability.

② The man places his hands on her hips and guides himself into her yoni. This is typically a very stimulating posture for the man, not only because of the angle of direct penetration but also because he can look down and watch the action. If she's flexible enough, she can look up and enjoy the action from a different angle.

③ To prolong enjoyment in this posture, he can slow his movements and take breaks to breathe and reach down to caress her breasts and abdomen. This can also give the woman a chance to be supported so she can bring her head up and enjoy the sensation of the increased blood flow to her head and upper body.

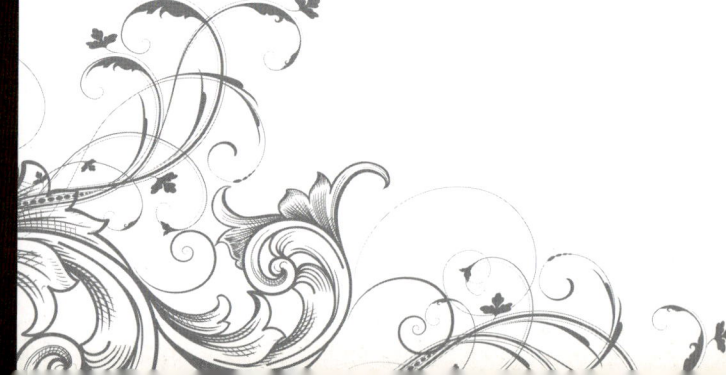

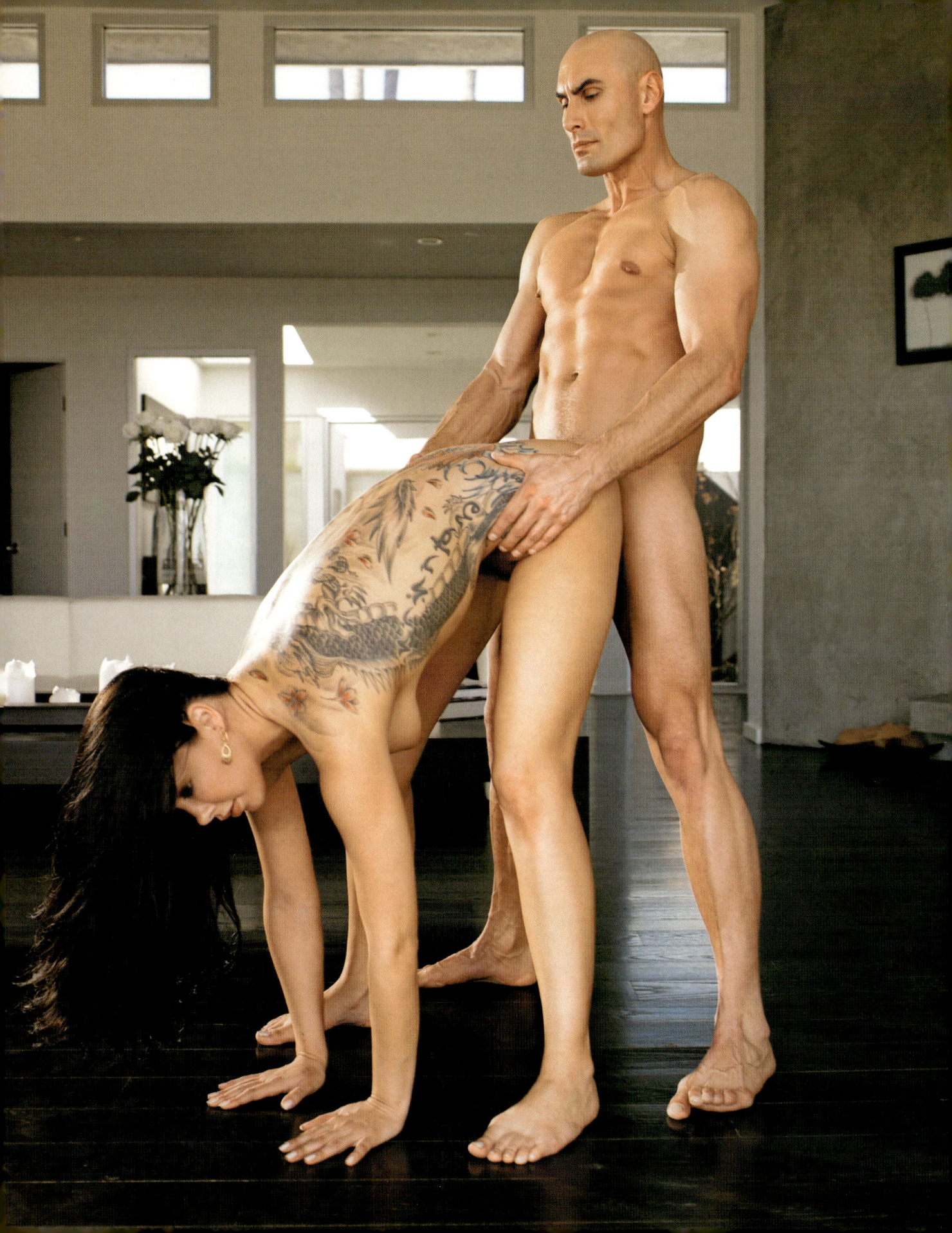

24 | CONGRESS OF A COW

{ A Variation of the Camel's Hump }

A POPULAR VARIATION of the Camel's Hump with a less-than-desirable name, this position is more relaxed, with the woman on all fours and the man kneeling behind her (or as it's described in the Kama Sutra, "her lover mounts her like a bull"). She can still arch her back up as in the Camel's Hump, but she can then do the opposite movement by throwing her head back, dropping her belly down, and swaying her back. Explore the different angles and pleasures to be had as she rotates her pelvis forward and backward in this way. He can hold on to her hips and practice a variety of thrusting methods: shallow, deep, slow, fast, to the right or left.

As an alternative for him, he can kneel on just one knee and place the other leg perpendicular to his body with his foot flat on the bed or floor. This can provide a different angle of penetration that may unleash new waves of orgasmic pleasure for you both.

As an alternative for her, she can come down to her elbows, resting her upper body on her forearms or leaning her chest on pillows with her cheek turned to the side. This will change the angle of penetration and may give her more direct stimulation on her G-spot.

> "Until sex is part of your complete self—including your spiritual self—you do not truly understand who you are."
>
> —*Deepak Chopra*, Kama Sutra

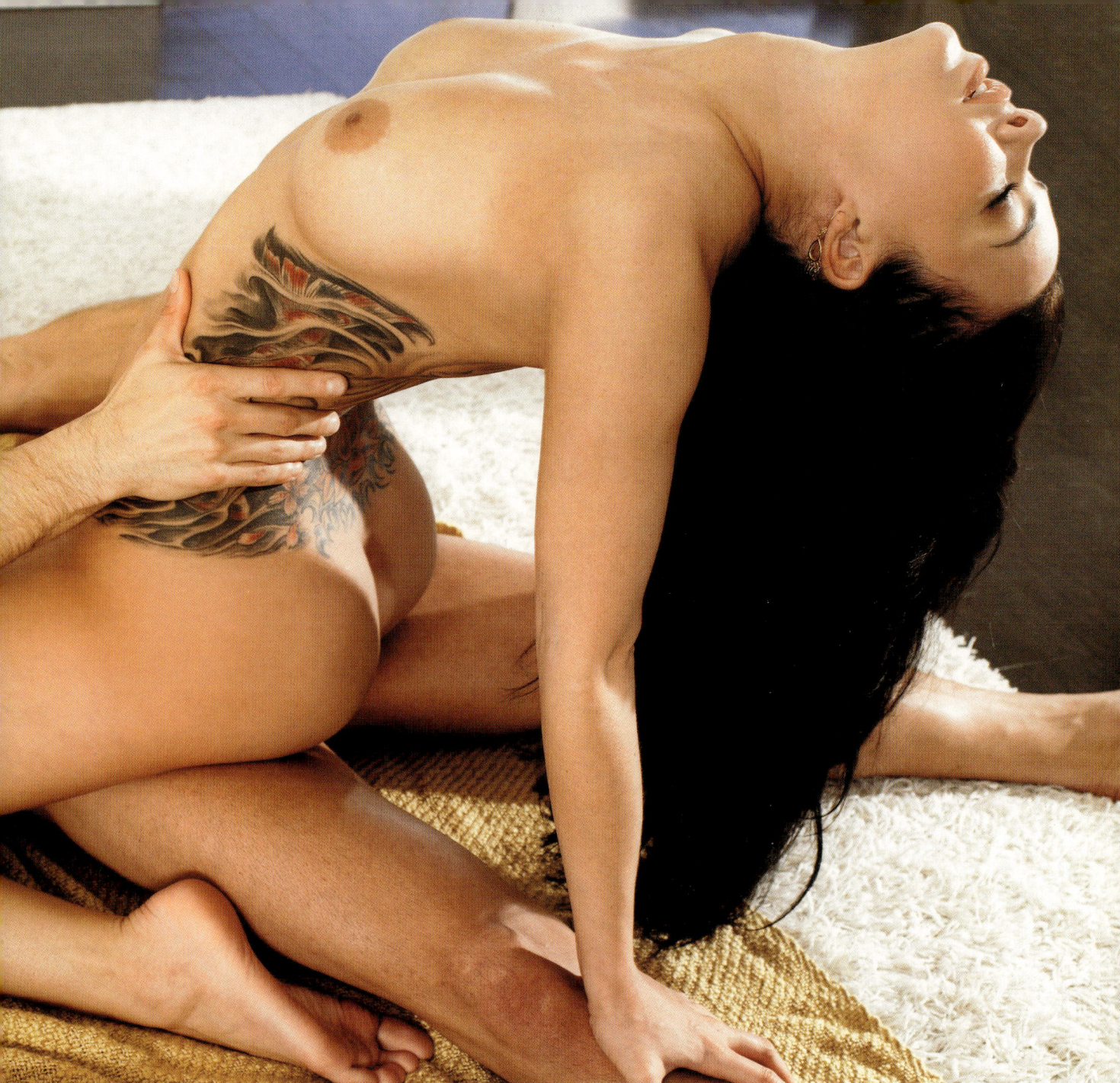

③ She then reaches back in a slight backbend and places her hands below his knees on his calves. Now she is free to tilt her head back sensually, exposing her neck and chest and allowing her hair to hang down freely. This is not a position of up and down penetration but rather a slow and sensual circular dance upon his vajra, like a belly dancer would do. The circular motion stimulates sexual energy and Shakti, the sacred feminine life force. The woman can play with both clockwise and counterclockwise directions as well as use the Love Pump squeeze internally to "suck" on his vajra and heighten her own orgasmic energy.

26 | SPLITTING THE BAMBOO

⟨ Playing His Bamboo Flute ⟩

IN ONE OF THE CLASSIC Kama Sutra positions, the woman alternately splits her legs, bending and straightening them. In this way, she creates a tightening sensation on his vajra and pleasurable friction for both lovers. The woman creates the movement in this posture, finding the ideal rhythm for them both. The man remains still and practices receiving while enjoying the show of his lover playing his "bamboo flute."

① The woman lies on her back with her hips raised up slightly on pillows. She brings both of her knees to her chest, exposing her yoni to her lover.

② He kneels in front of her and enters her, opening his knees wide and placing them on either side of her hips. To give her freedom to move her legs, he can bring his arms up, interlace his hands, and clasp them behind his neck. Alternatively, he can place his hands on the small of his back or gently hold on to her body and switch up his grip as she moves her legs. She grasps his thighs to support her movement.

③ She leaves one leg down and stretches the other one out straight behind him. Then she alternates, bending the straightened leg while straightening her other leg. This will be a good abdominal workout for the woman.

④ If she gets tired alternating her legs, the man can take over the rhythm and gently thrust for a while until she's ready to switch leg positions again. She can also use her internal muscles to massage his erection and generate more orgasmic energy for them both.

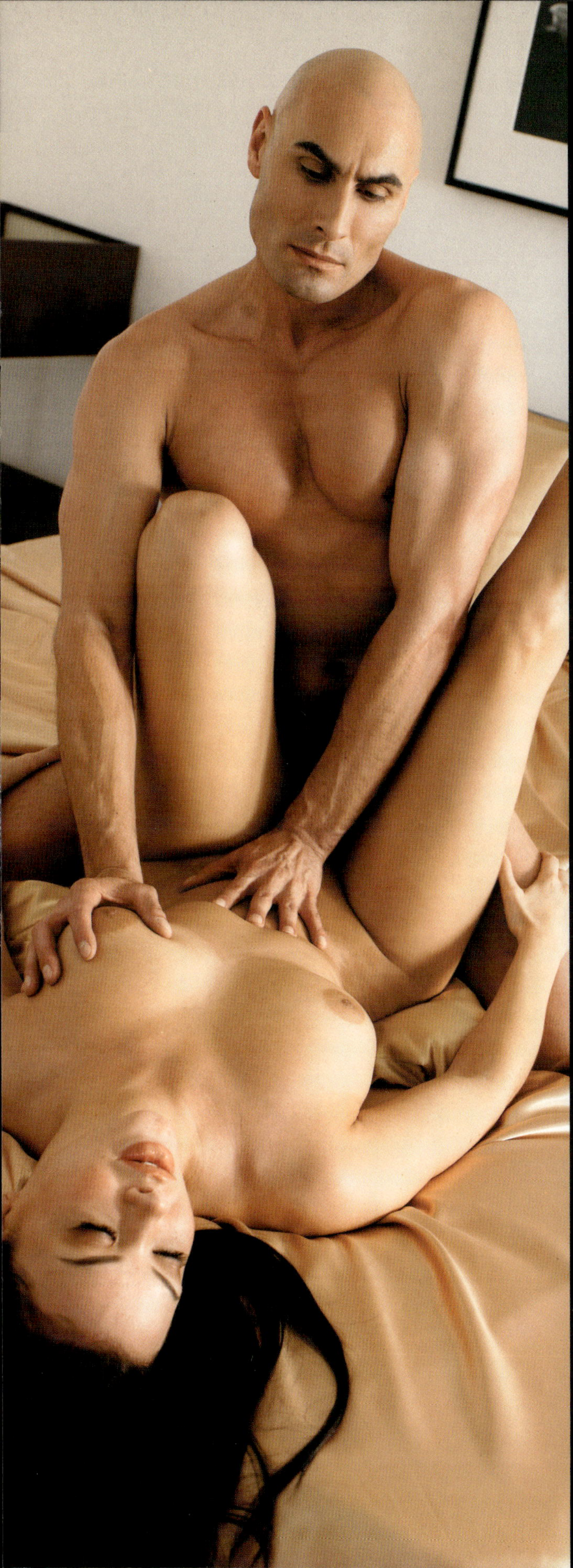

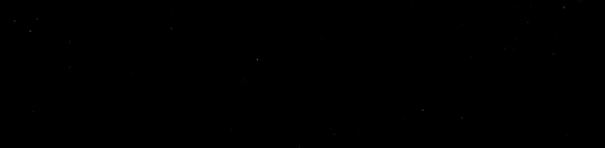

The Art of Kissing

Perhaps the Kama Sutra has endured throughout the ages because it so thoroughly addresses the full spectrum of lovemaking, not just the positions. And nothing has the power to kindle the fire of passion like a kiss. Vatsyayana meticulously describes many types of kisses, including "nominal, throbbing, touching, straight, bent, turned, pressed, clasping, and wrestling tongue."

Because it's likely that you've been kissing for a while now, use this list to inspire some creativity. Maybe you're in a rut and noticing that your kisses don't seem to make her knees weak anymore or light a fire in his eyes. Worse yet—maybe you've stopped kissing altogether!

Remember your first kisses and how terribly exciting they were? Remember kissing for hours, just because it felt so good? If your kissing has become boring, or merely a perfunctory stop on the way to something "more exciting," it's time to re-evaluate. Start fresh, with "beginner's mind," and rediscover what you've been missing.

Here's a practice: Let one partner give the kiss while the other receives it. Then switch. If you're receiving, totally relax your mouth and let your lover explore. No kissing back! If you're kissing a woman, use your tongue to stimulate the spot between the inside of her upper lip and her gum line, right in the center. Tantric teachings note a connection between this spot and a woman's clitoris. When kissing a man, run your tongue along the opposite spot, between the inside of his lower lip and gum in the center. This point is said to stimulate the frenulum, or delicate tissue underneath the head of his vajra.

27 | THE SWING

{ You'll Fly in This Sitting Position }

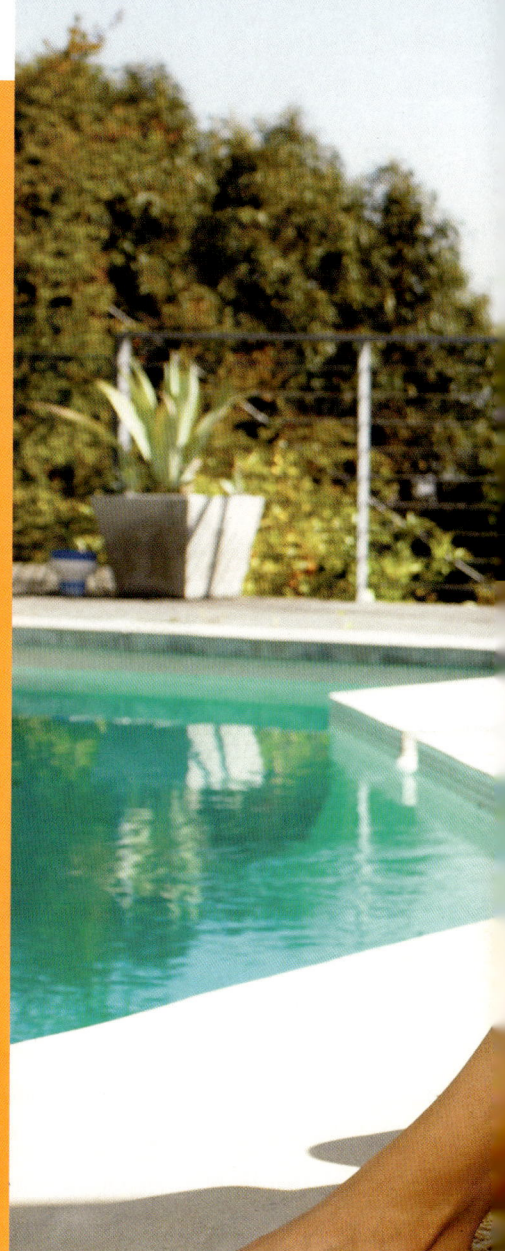

WITH BOTH LOVERS holding and supporting one another, this sitting position encourages prolonged lovemaking by making it easy to alternate between times of passionate energy and relaxation. Facing one another gives you the opportunity to build intimacy through eye contact as well as to kiss each other deeply. Because the woman has a great deal of control over the depth and speed of penetration and can easily stimulate her clitoris, this can be a very orgasmic position for her.

① The man sits on a firm surface with his legs outstretched. A pillow or cushion under his butt will make him most comfortable, particularly for a longer lovemaking session.

② The woman sits between his legs, resting her weight partially on his thighs as she places his vajra inside her and wraps one arm around her lover's shoulders. She can place her other arm around his shoulder as well or, for more leverage, she can place it on the floor behind her or hold on to his thigh. Her legs are open with either her toes or feet about hip-distance apart on the floor behind him.

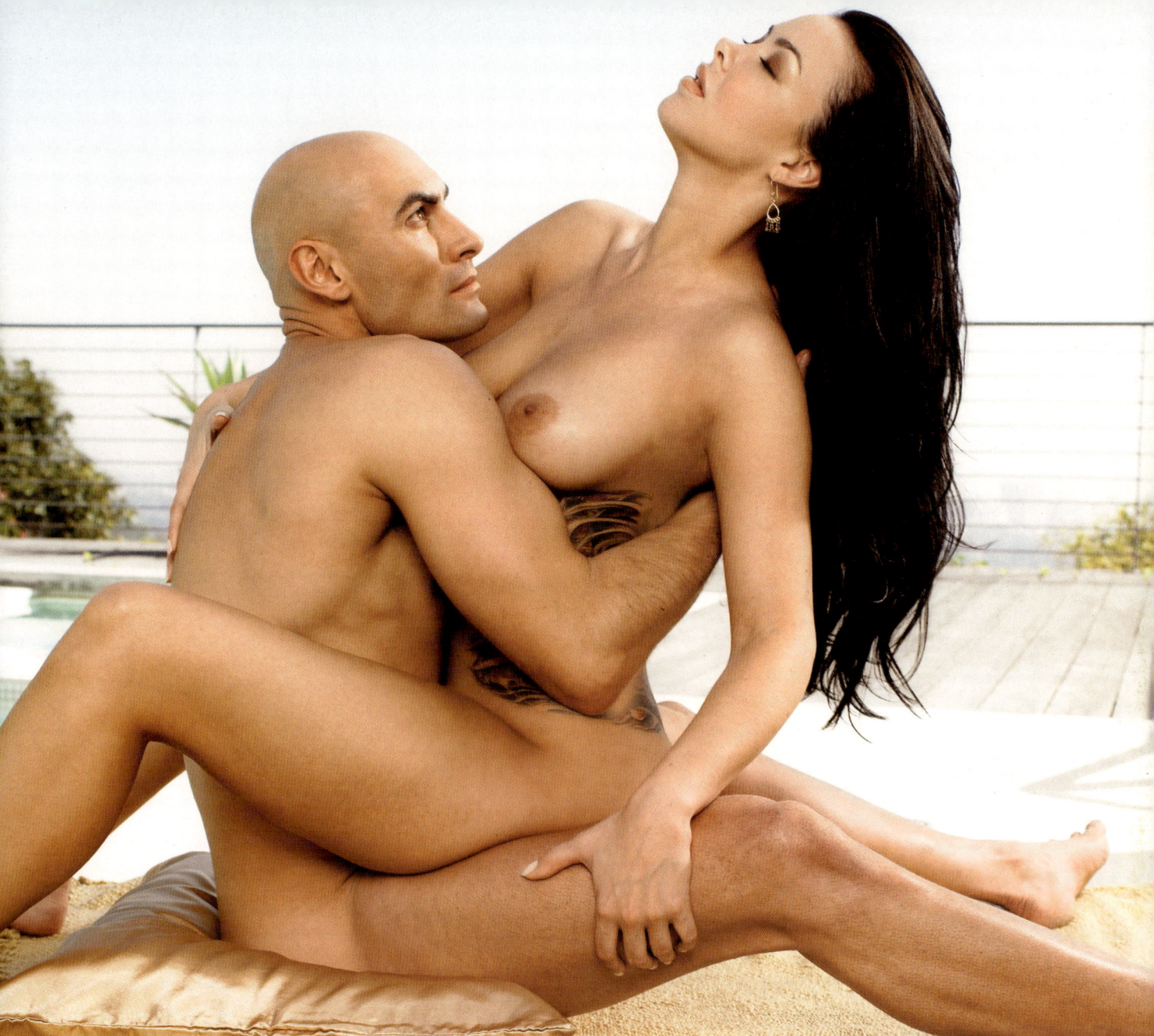

③ He wraps his arms around her back to support her. To "dial in" the right angle between her yoni and his vajra or to offer more support to the woman and less pressure on the lap of the man, consider folding a firm pillow in half and placing it long side up underneath her.

④ Once in the position, use the weight of your bodies to "swing" back and forth, finding a natural rhythm that brings you maximum pleasure. As the woman swings, she can arch her back, which opens her heart, and she can let her hair fall behind her as if it were flowing in the wind. By mutually supporting one another, you can enjoy this swinging rhythm as you ride waves of increasing pleasure.

28 | THE SWAN

{ Reverse Cowboy, Kama Sutra Style }

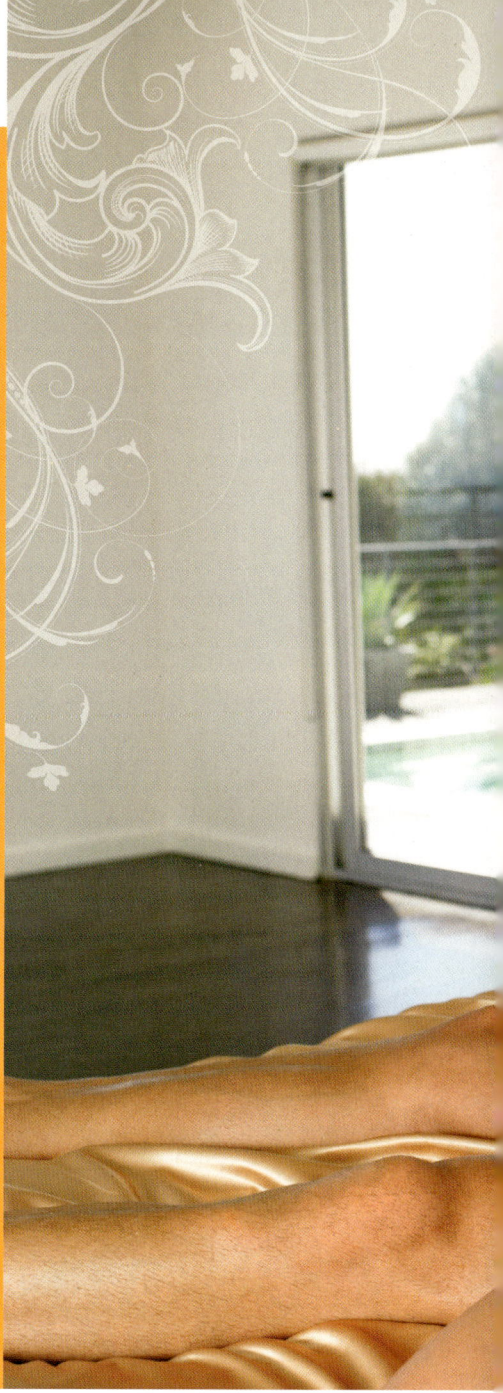

IN THIS COMBINATION woman-on-top and rear-entry position, the graceful arc of the woman's hips and back echo that of a swan. By not facing each other, you have the opportunity to tune in more deeply to your individual body sensations. Because of the angle of penetration, the woman can experience stimulation in new areas of her yoni. The position also tends to pull his vajra down somewhat, which can heighten sensation for the man.

As in other women-on-top positions, this one allows a woman to easily reach her clitoris and fondle her breasts or nipples while the man gets to enjoy the view and hold her butt. If you're a woman who feels self-conscious being watched while you self-pleasure, then this is a good beginner pose because it gives you some privacy while still being connected to your partner. If it is challenging for you to reach orgasm through intercourse (which is common for many women), then being able to bring yourself to orgasm in this position with your man inside you will help "teach" your body how to do it in other positions. Once your body gets the hang of it, it becomes easier and easier.

① The man lies on his back with his legs stretched out and close together. The woman kneels beside him, straddles him on her knees facing his feet, and lowers herself onto his vajra. Alternately, she can stand over him with her feet on either side of his hips and squat down, lowering herself onto him and then coming to her knees.

② She can flex her yoni muscles in a Love Pump to stimulate them both. She can rock back and forth or move in a circular motion as well. She does the work in this position while he gets to admire her sensual movements on his erection.

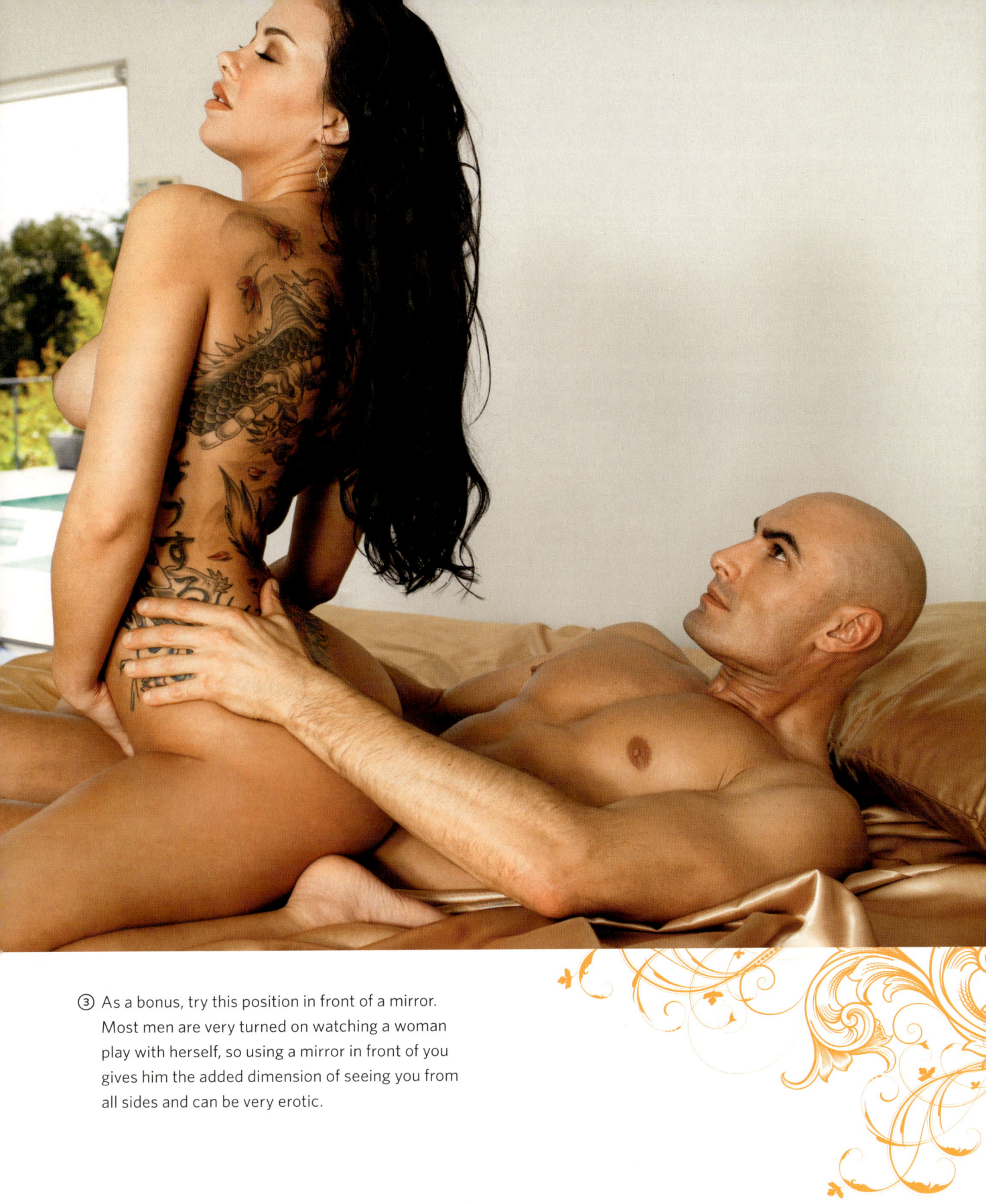

③ As a bonus, try this position in front of a mirror. Most men are very turned on watching a woman play with herself, so using a mirror in front of you gives him the added dimension of seeing you from all sides and can be very erotic.

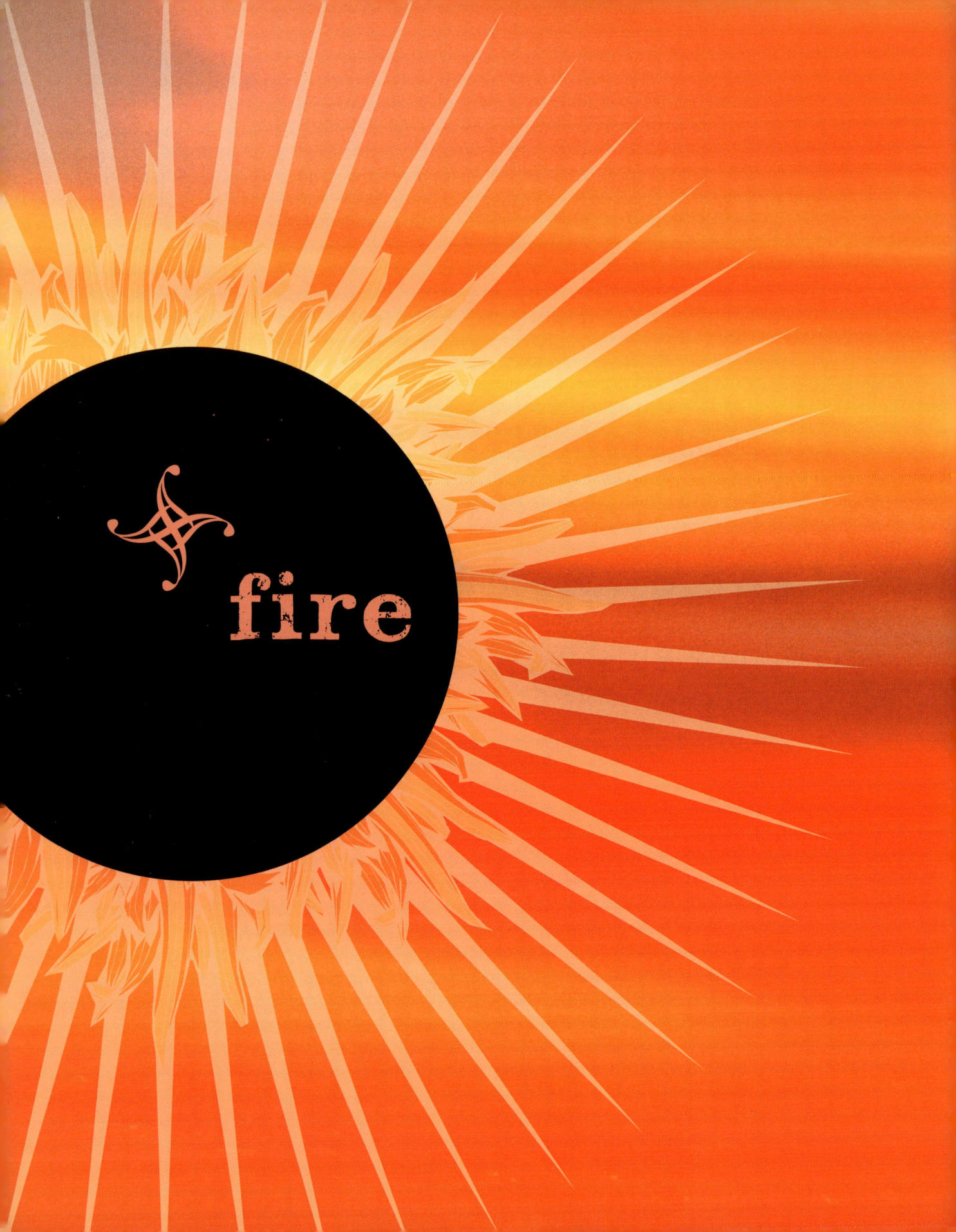

fire

THERE'S NO EXTINGUISHING THE FIRE NOW. THE PASSION BLAZES WITH A FOCUSED INTENSITY AND ABANDON. IT GATHERS STRENGTH AND DANCES ON THE EDGE OF CONTROL, PULSING WITH HEAT, MELTING RESISTANCE INTO A MOLTEN "YES, YES, YES." BURN IT UP WITH THESE KAMA SUTRA POSTURES DESIGNED FOR LOVERS WHO WANT TO SPICE IT UP AND GET MORE PHYSICAL.

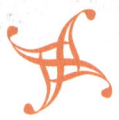

29 | SHAKTI

{ The Woman's on Top and in Control }

THE ANCIENT TANTRIC MASTERS believed that all creation came from the erotic union of the great god Shiva and his consort Shakti, representing pure life force and the divine feminine principle. In this position, the woman allows herself to embody her sacred feminine power.

At her core, the feminine wants to be looked at and seen (maybe it's why we love to dress up and need so *many* pairs of shoes). At his core, the masculine wants and needs to look (so *maybe* he's not being a jerk when his eye wanders). In this position, the man gets to watch and she gets to be seen. It can be even more erotic when she self-pleasures and allows herself to be witnessed openly feeling her own orgasmic energy.

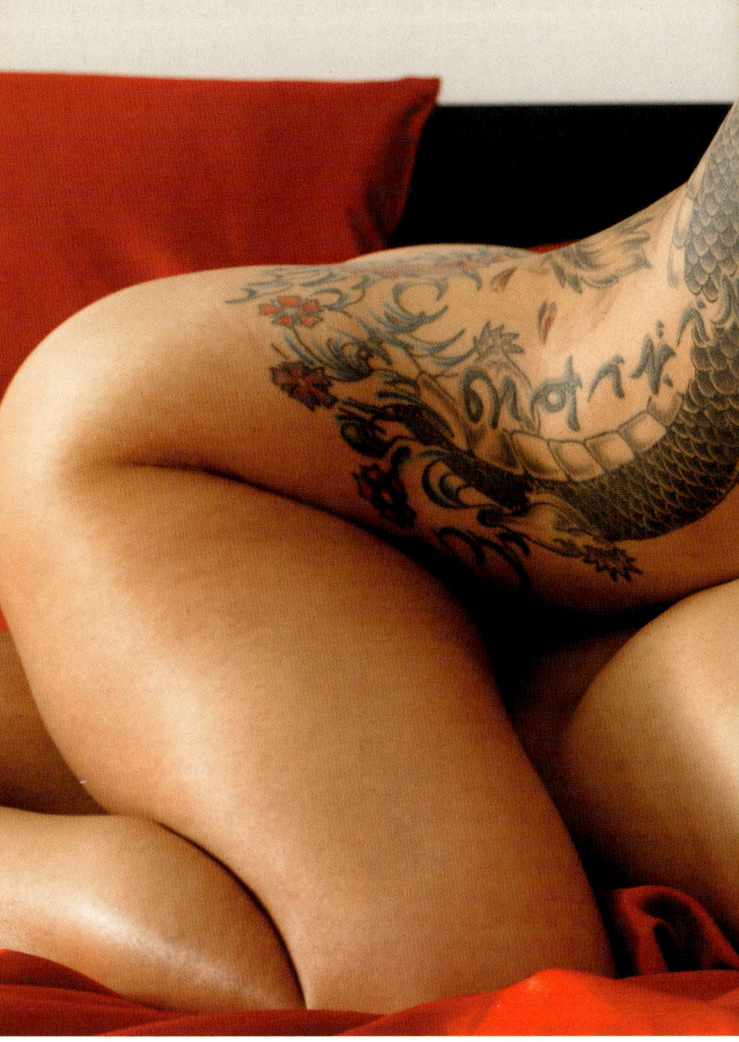

① Start by making the man comfortable on his back. The woman begins to tease and arouse him. Drag your hair and breasts over his entire body. Kiss him up and down. Crawl around on him. Smell and taste him.

② When it's time for penetration, the woman straddles the man and lifts herself up onto her knees as much as necessary to mount him. Sitting upright, she can grind in slow, sensual circles on his vajra, ride him forward and backward, or stay outwardly still and use the Love Pump. Because she's in control of the movement, she's in an ideal position to find just the right angle to stimulate her G-spot.

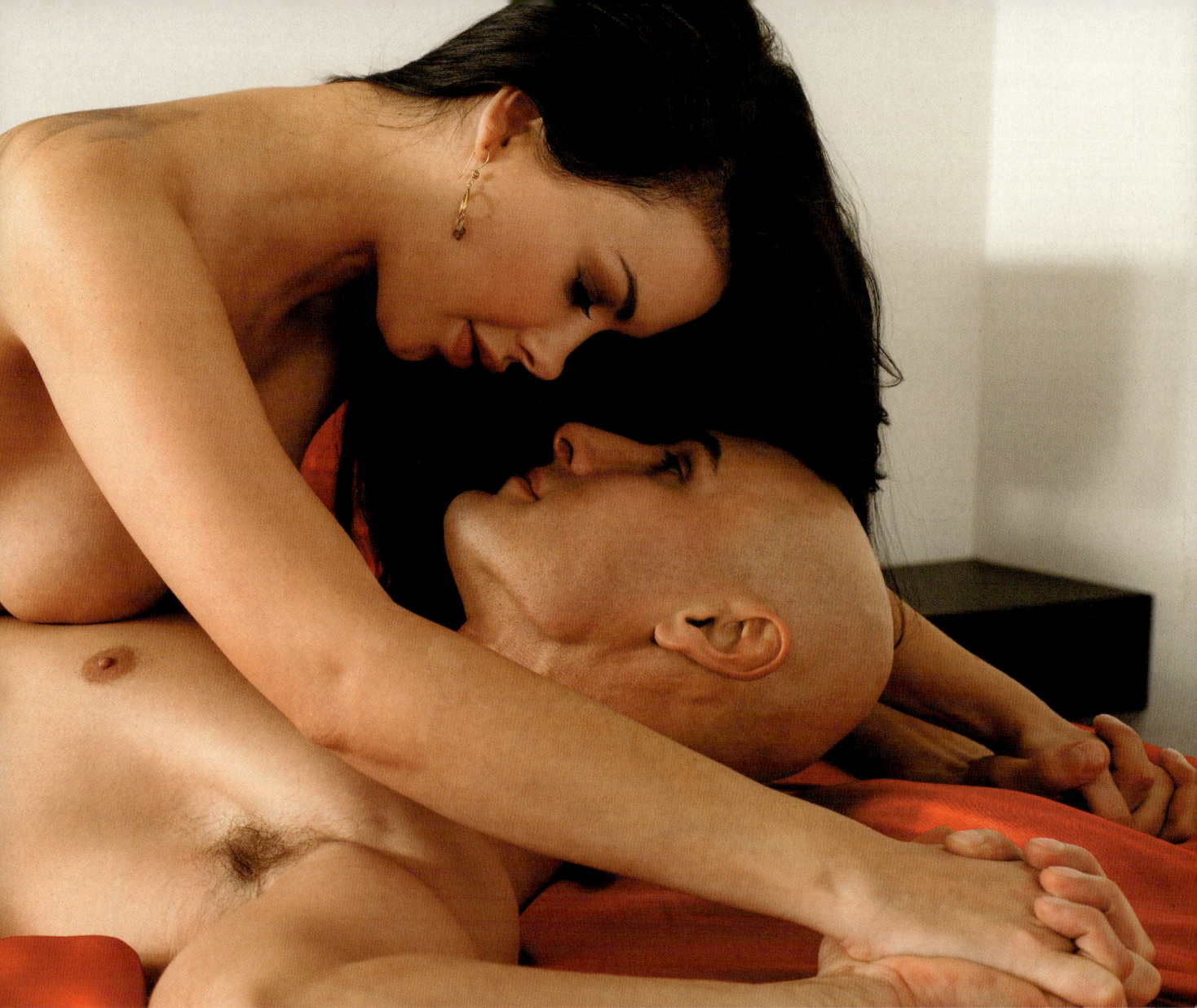

③ As an alternative, she can place her feet flat on either side of his hips and squat down on top of him. In this position, she can use her leg muscles to pump up and down on his vajra and give him the sensation of no part of her body touching him except her yoni.

④ She can also try laying her entire body down on his so they can be heart to heart. The man can either fully surrender to the movements of the woman or he can tilt his pelvis forward in a thrusting motion to meet her rhythm as well. She can explore her "inner tiger" by interlacing her fingers with his and pressing them above his head as she "pins" him with her loving passion.

30 | THE TONGS

{ *Grip His Vajra with Your Tongs* }

THIS IS ONE OF SEVERAL WOMAN-ON-TOP positions that Vatsyayana recommended as a good alternative if a man becomes fatigued and needs a break during lovemaking. The pleasure will depend on the woman having a strong Love Pump so that she can internally suck, pulse, and grip his vajra like a pair of tongs, ideally for " a hundred heartbeats." Because the action happens internally and the couple remains relatively motionless externally, it can also be an excellent position for the adventurous couple who wants to make love outdoors without drawing attention—a strategically placed beach blanket can do the trick.

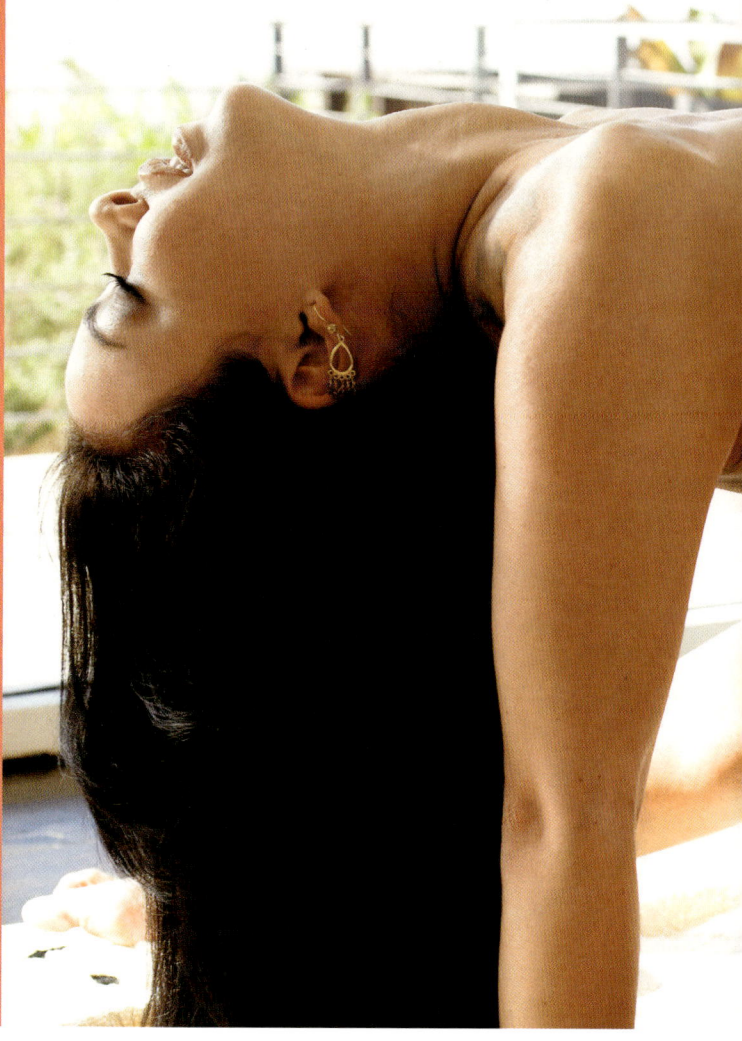

① The man sits with his legs out and the woman mounts him in a straddle, keeping her legs apart and her feet on the ground for support. You both lean away from each other slightly, she resting on outstretched arms while he holds her gently around the waist for support. He can lean against a bolster or a small piece of furniture as well to support his back. As you both lean back, you'll notice that the penetration can be very deep, but the man does no thrusting.

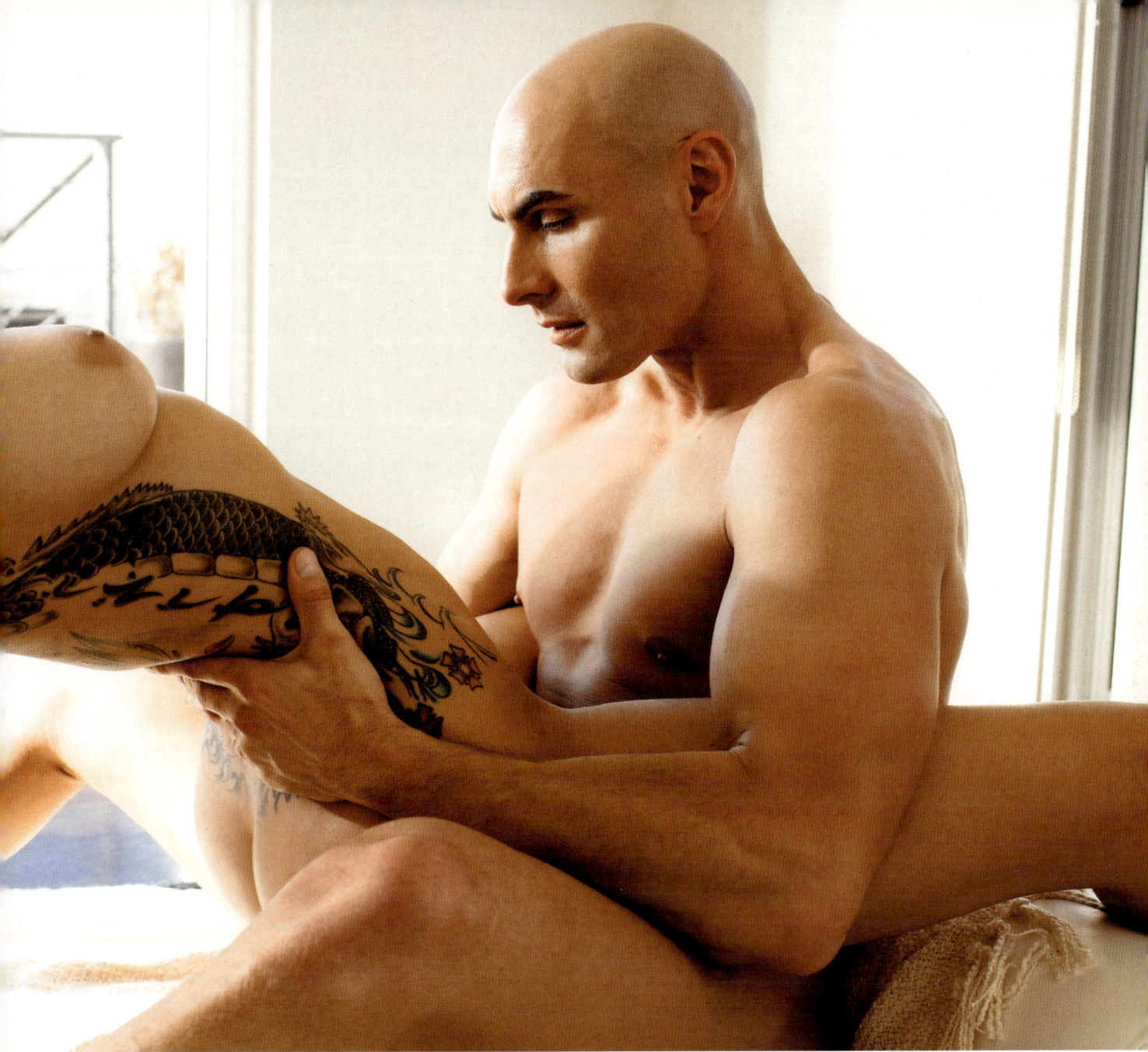

② The woman then flexes her love muscle internally while they both remain still on the outside. She can begin by slowly squeezing as she inhales to a count of six and then releasing the muscles on the exhalation. She can also try small, rapid pulsations, almost like fluttering butterfly wings. Experiment with different ways of stroking, caressing, and undulating your muscles to find what brings you both the most pleasure. If you're used to vigorous sex, you'll need to have patience as you train your genitals to have greater awareness and enjoyment with more subtle sensations. As you do, you may be surprised when you're rewarded with possibly even more intense and longer orgasms than you ever experienced in more athletic positions.

31 | SINGING MONKEY

{ The Woman's on Top of Her Seated Man }

UNLESS YOU HAPPEN TO HAVE
a straight-backed chair in your boudoir, this
woman-on-top position may encourage you to
venture outside of the bedroom for some passionate lovemaking in the dining room or outside (or
even the boardroom at the office!). A change of
scenery can help you break out of stuck patterns,
bringing you more fully into the "now" with you
partner—always a powerful aphrodisiac.

> "Yes, it's true that the senses can lead
> you astray and the pursuit of pleasure
> can get you in trouble. Sensual pleasure
> needs the guidance of practical and
> ethical judgment. But you won't gain
> good health by repeatedly vetoing the
> vote of the senses and denigrating
> the wisdom of the body. Nature was
> neither capricious nor perverted in
> making sure that, other things being
> equal, what feels good is good for you."
>
> —*George Leonard, Author*

① The man sits comfortably on a straight-backed
chair with his feet firmly on the ground and his
knees slightly apart.

② The woman approaches him at whatever speed
she desires. She may choose to go slowly,
perhaps seductively removing her clothing or
undressing as she approaches him. She may
dance for him, sway her hips, or touch herself
sensually while she maintains eye contact with
her lover, building the desire and anticipation.
Alternately, you may both be full of fire and
intensity, and this is a great position for an
immediate, passionate connection. The woman
can quickly straddle her man, wrap her hands
behind his neck, and be in full torso contact while
kissing him deeply.

③ Depending on the height of both the woman and
the chair, she may have her feet flat on the floor,
be elevated on her toes, or use the bottom rung
of the chair for balance. The more traction she
has, the more range of motion and control she
will have in the position. With a lot of stability,
she has the option of rotating her hips in circles,
rocking back and forth, and even raising and
lowering herself onto his erection. If she is up on
her toes, her partner can take charge of the
balance and intensity by holding her butt and
either thrusting from his seated position or lifting
her up and down simultaneously.

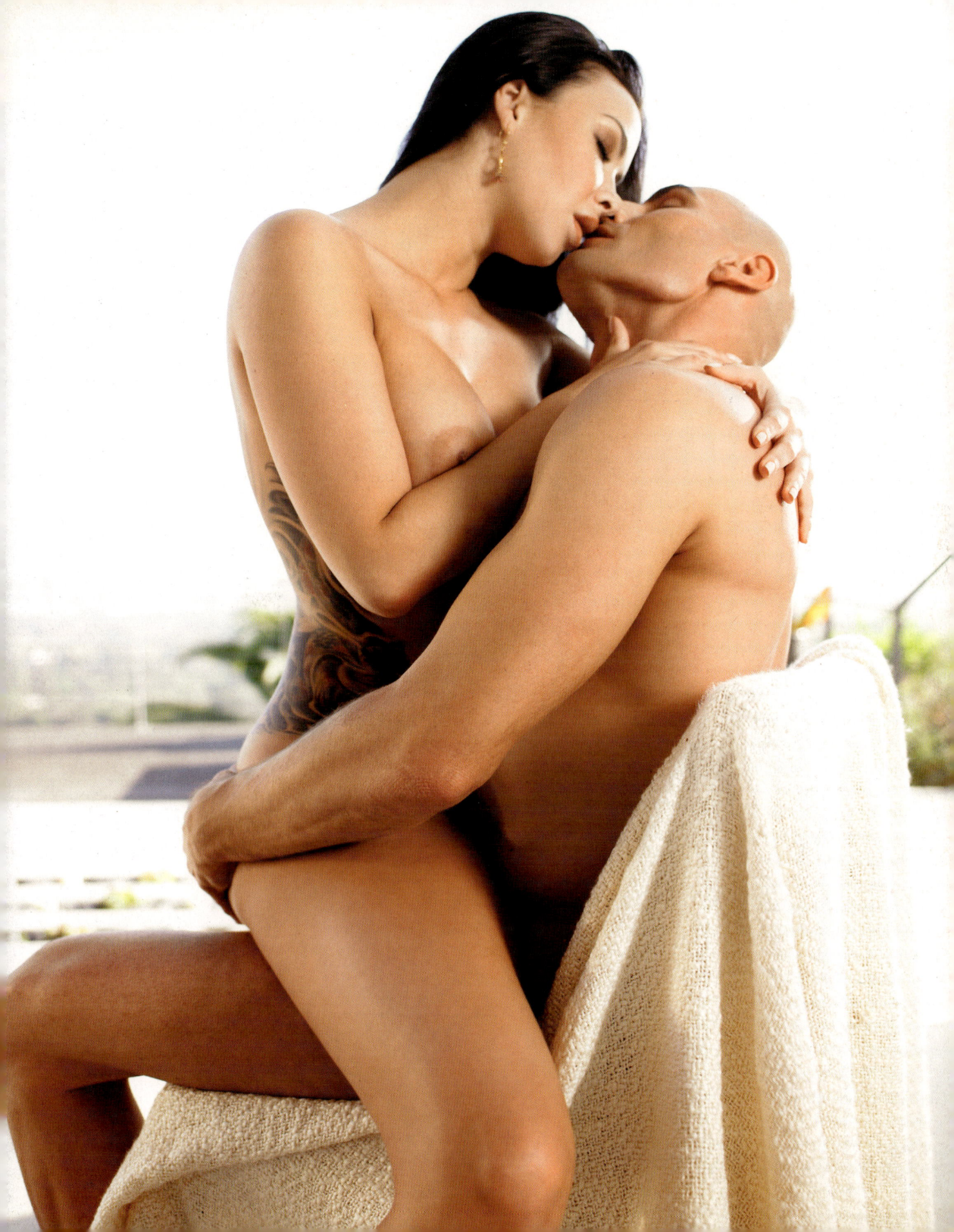

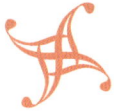

32 | SULTAN

{ He'll Be Enslaved by Desire }

WHEN WE SWITCH UP the roles we usually play in lovemaking, we discover new things about ourselves and our partners. Without old patterns, we land more fully in the present, where any number of erotic delights may surprise us. In this position, the man takes the passive role, literally on his back with his knees apart, while the woman takes control of the action. He is treated like a great sultan who is being pleasured by his favorite courtesan.

① The woman sits upright on the bed with her legs open wide and her knees bent slightly. With outstretched arms, she invites her man to come into her loving embrace. He sits facing her with his legs bent and placed over hers, if possible touching the soles of his feet together behind her.

② Placing her feet flat and firmly on the bed to support herself, the woman scoots as close as possible to him, rocking gently. He places his arms loosely around her, allowing himself to be held and relaxing his head on her shoulder. This can be a rejuvenating posture for a man after an intense day and, as she rocks and presses her breasts and pelvis rhythmically against him, it can bring them both into heightened arousal.

③ Next the woman encourages him to lie back slowly by gradually supporting his arms and assisting him onto a nest of pillows fit for a king. Here he can completely relax and be pampered while she strokes his legs and vajra, whispering words of appreciation and love.

④ When they are both aroused, she slowly bends her legs behind her, coming up onto her knees and pressing her pelvis toward him. She can also put her feet flat on the bed or floor and come into a squatting position over him. She brings his knees up and presses them open, exposing him fully. From this position, she tilts her pelvis forward and guides his vajra into her. She gently bounces and presses into him, holding on to his legs for leverage. This can be a very empowering and erotic position for women, who may delight in the sensation of thrusting for a change. Men can feel liberated being so open and surrendered.

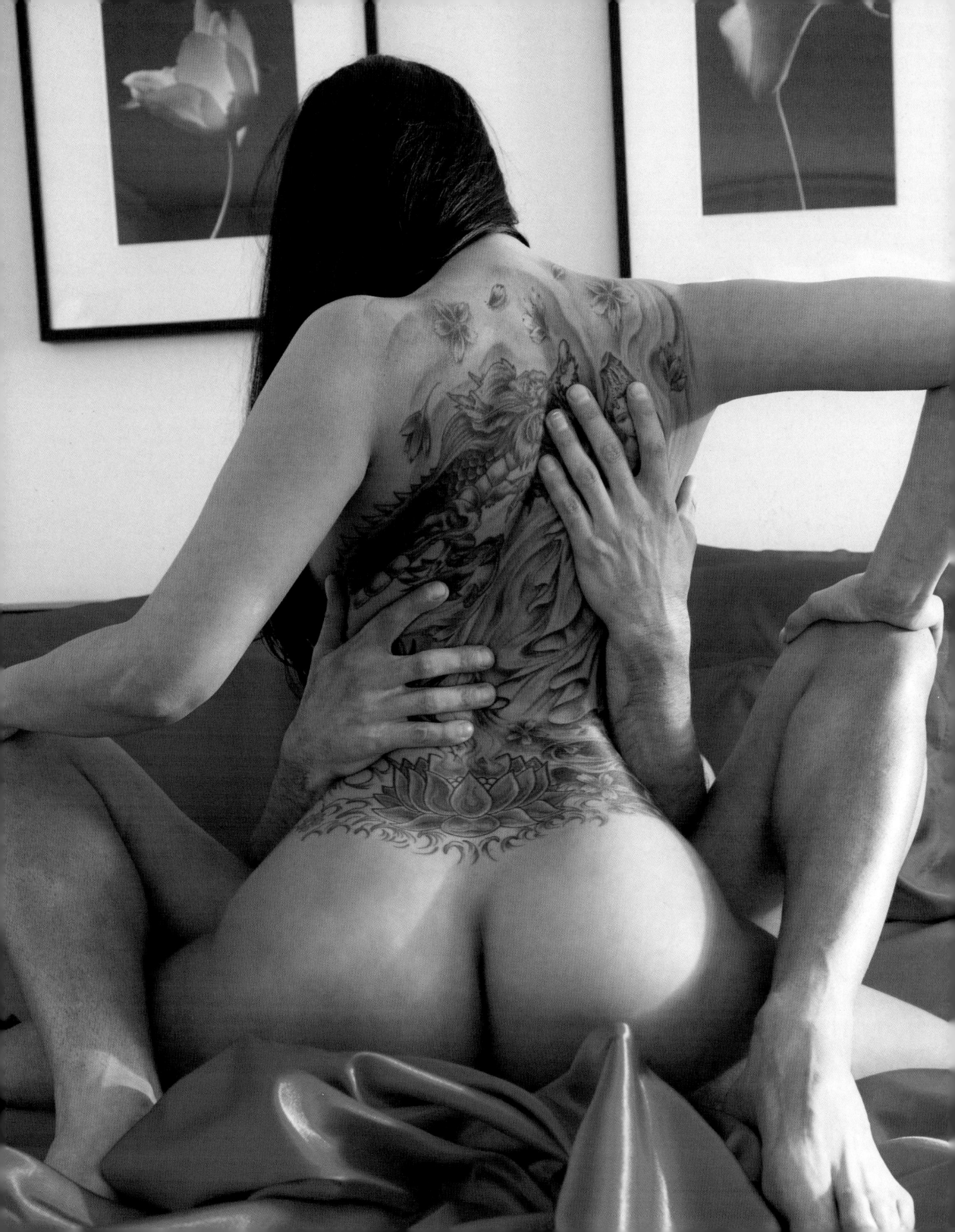

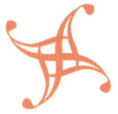

33 | RAJA

❧ Bonded Together in Abandon ❧

IN THE BEGINNING stage of this posture, you'll come into harmony with one another in an intimate embrace where the man lovingly holds the woman in his lap and you enjoy the erotic sensation from the pressure of your genitals together. The final expression will be most rewarding for a woman with some yoga experience and open, flexible hips.

① The man sits upright with his legs out in front of him. She sits sideways on his lap with her right leg crossed over her left, keeping her knees and feet together. She bends her knees and tucks her feet behind him so that they hold him. Her right arm circles his left shoulder, and she can place her left arm behind her for balance. His right arm can hold her tucked legs while he circles her waist with his left hand, using upper body strength to pull her close.

② Spend time soul gazing, basking in the embrace, and feeling the delight of your genitals pressed together. This can also be an ideal position for the man to kiss and pleasure the woman's breasts to build arousal. When you're both ready for intercourse, she can lean away from him while he places his vajra inside her.

③ For the more advanced expression of the posture, the woman places her outstretched left arm below his right knee for leverage and slowly, gracefully lifts her right leg up high, crossing it in front of his face to rest the back of her right knee on top of his left shoulder. She places her left foot flat on the bed or floor behind him for balance, and they wrap their arms around each other. Although this posture provides little room for external movement, it offers a deep and healing pelvic opening for the woman, and strong bonding for the couple. She can also practice the Love Pump (page 69) to massage his vajra and generate orgasmic energy.

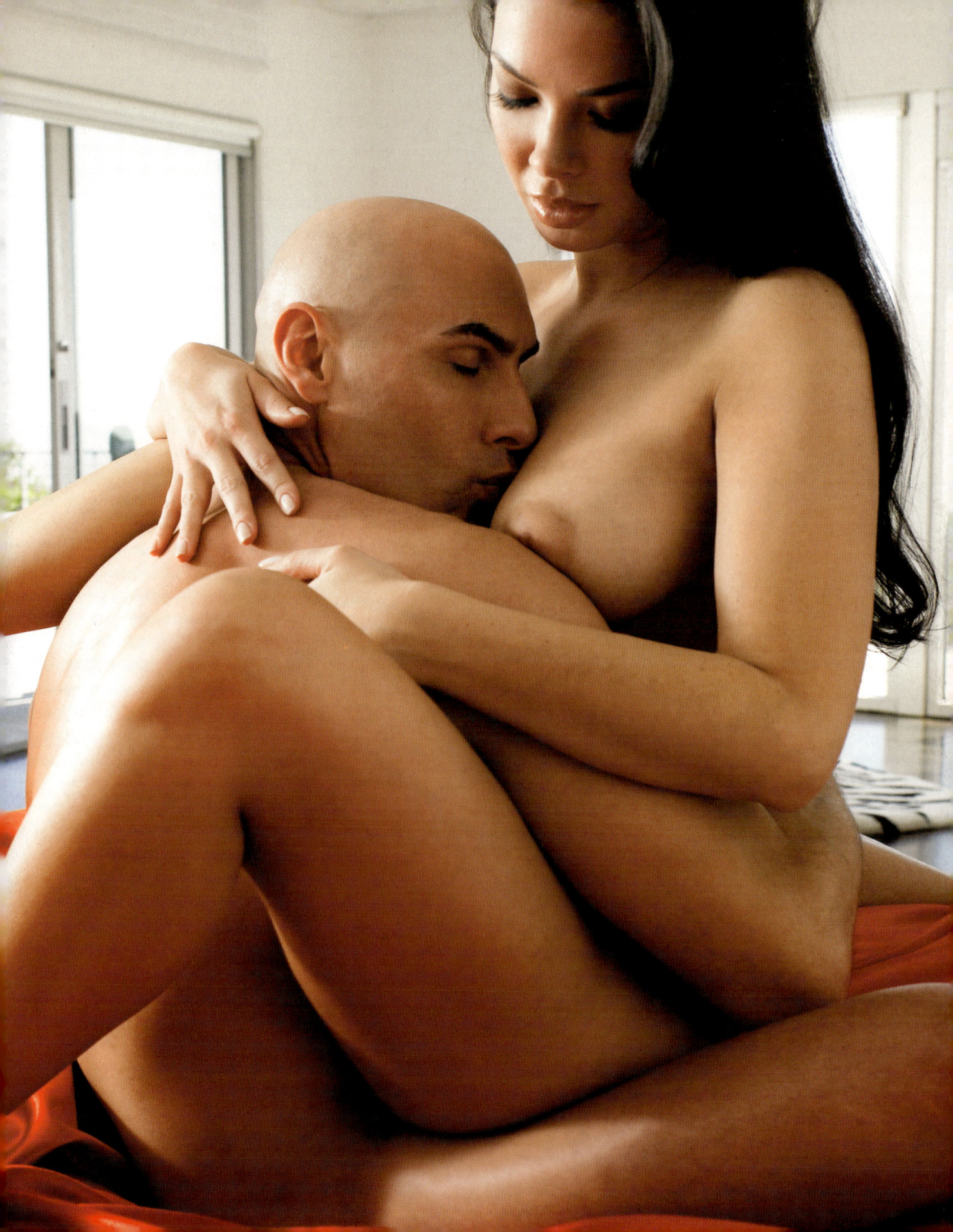

34 | DIAMOND

{ A Brilliant Pelvic Connection }

THIS VISUALLY BEAUTIFUL posture will help bring you into balance inside yourself and with your partner. It powerfully opens and expands the heart, so try it when your relationship needs a boost of harmonic convergence. Remember the feeling of the wind rushing through your hair as you leaned back in total abandonment as a kid on the swings? Use this position to let go like that with your lover.

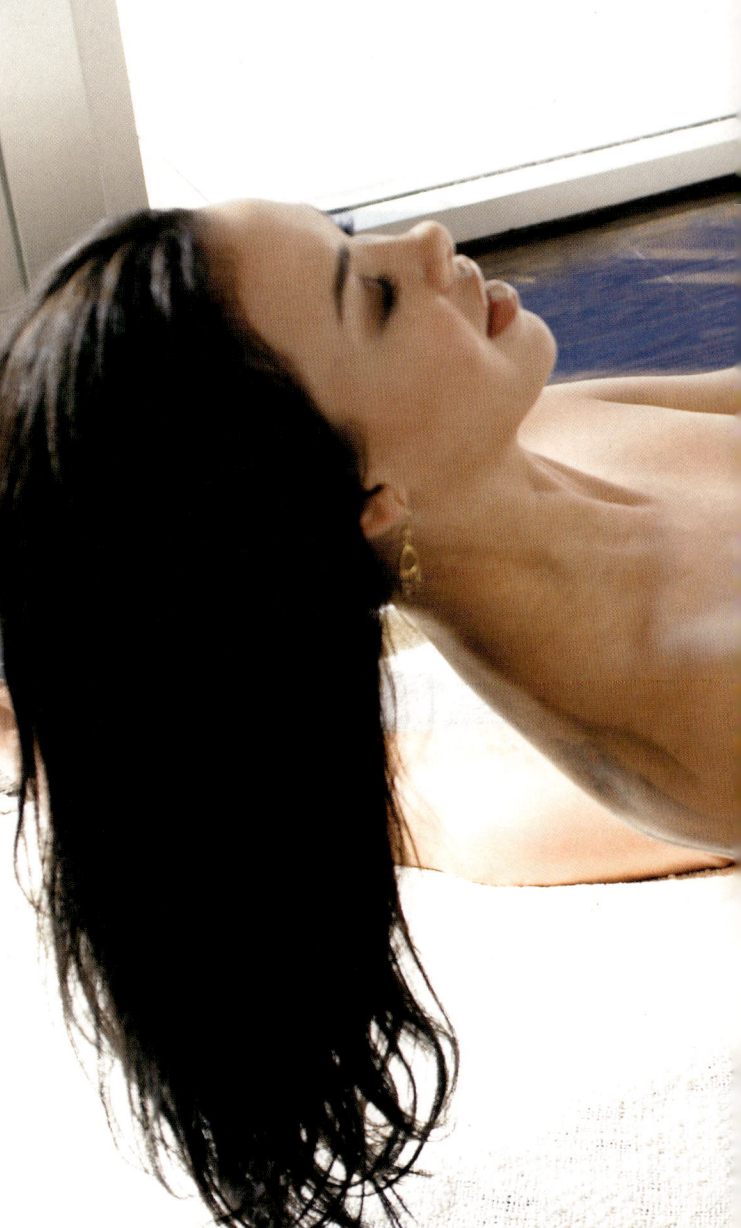

① Sit facing each other and come into harmony with your breath as you gaze at one other. This is an ideal time to do the Heart Salutation (see page 41) as a way to bring yourself into present with one another and call forth your sacred sexual energy.

② Next, the man opens his legs and stretches them out straight. The woman does the same, placing her legs on top of his and pressing her yoni against his vajra (which should be placed "up"). Stroke and caress one another, building the sexual energy.

③ When you're both ready, the woman raises herself up and lowers herself onto his erection. The movements here are internal: She uses her yoni muscles to massage his vajra. He uses his Love Pump to gently flex inside her.

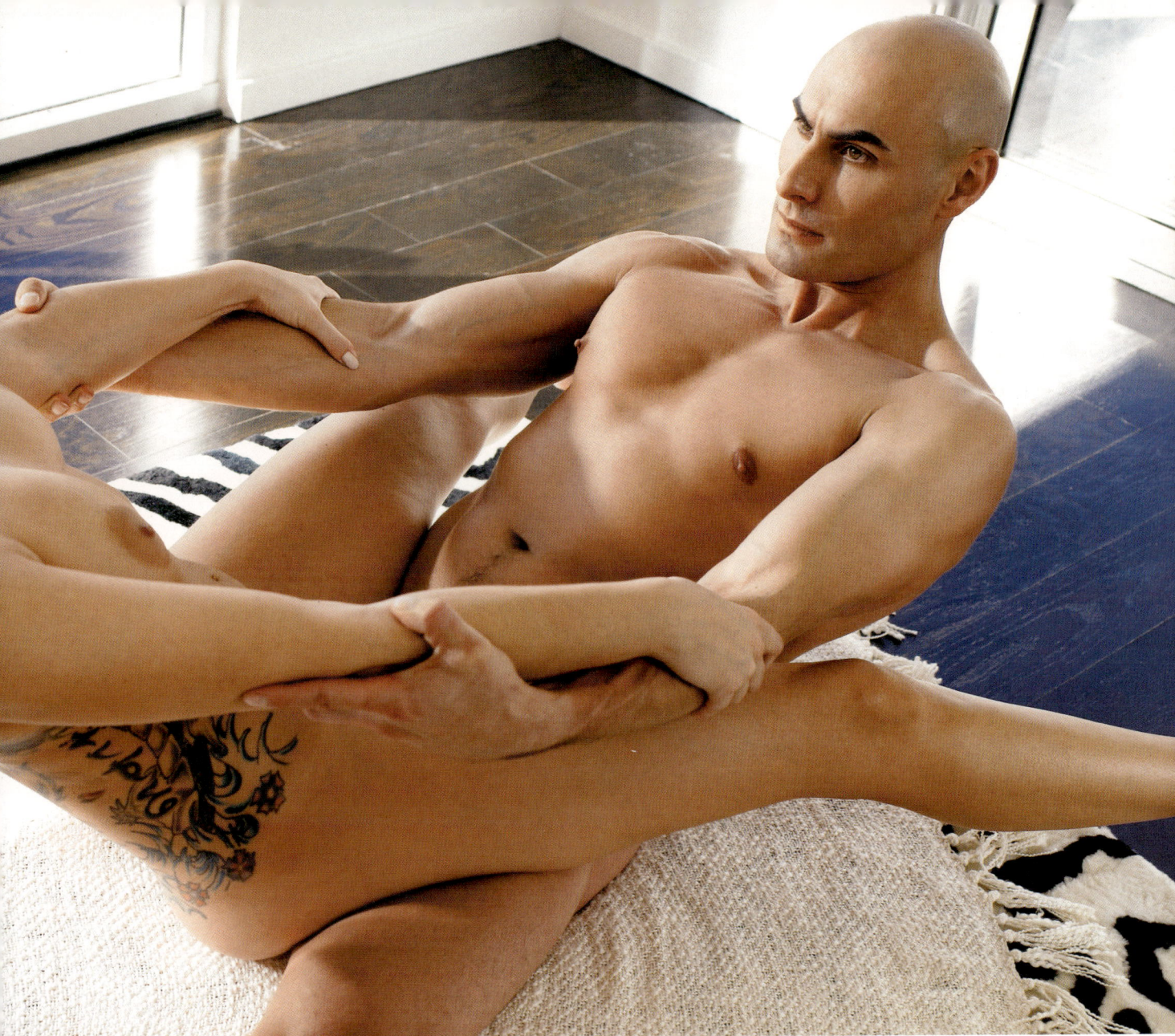

④ As your orgasmic energy builds, hold hands and find the point where you can both lean back, comfortably counterbalanced. To vary the angle of penetration and the depth of the backbend, you can also grasp each other around the wrist or forearm. Feel your heart opening as you relax your head back and close your eyes. Enjoy the depth of pleasure you feel with the concentration of so much energy in the pelvis and the rest of your body barely touching. Looking from above, your bodies make the shape of a perfect diamond, sparkling with light.

⑤ Inhaling together, draw the orgasmic energy up from your pelvis and into your heart. Exhale the sexual energy down your arms and out your hands. Visualize it entering into the hands of your beloved and traveling down his body and into his pelvis, completing the circuit between you. Practicing this way will help you achieve more expansive states of orgasmic bliss and oneness, the real "jewel" of your lovemaking.

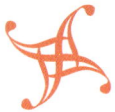

35 | RIDING THE ELEPHANT

{ Great Things Come in Small Places }

THIS COMPACT POSITION is ideal for an intimate connection in a very small place, such as in the canopy seat used by elephant riders. The rocking motion of the elephant also means very little movement is required, but do try this pleasurable position at home, even if you don't have access to an elephant.

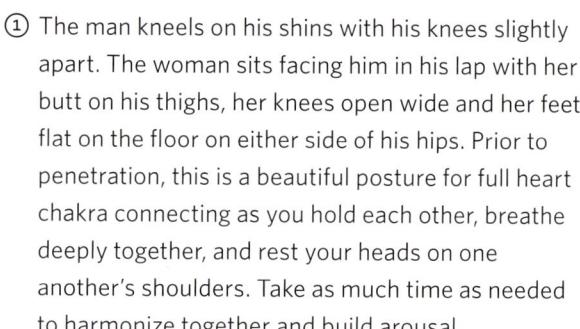

① The man kneels on his shins with his knees slightly apart. The woman sits facing him in his lap with her butt on his thighs, her knees open wide and her feet flat on the floor on either side of his hips. Prior to penetration, this is a beautiful posture for full heart chakra connecting as you hold each other, breathe deeply together, and rest your heads on one another's shoulders. Take as much time as needed to harmonize together and build arousal.

② When ready, the man supports the woman by holding her hips as she uses her legs to rise up slightly and lower herself back down onto his vajra. After several breaths together and some time to integrate the feeling of penetration, the woman then twists her body slightly to the right, wrapping her right leg as snugly as possible around the man's butt. The man then twists slightly to his right so that he can reach comfortably behind him to grasp her right ankle. By pulling on her right leg, he can have some control over their movements together.

③ With his left hand, he can hold her butt firmly, assisting her to "ride the elephant." She can support herself with her left hand on his side or hold him around his back with both arms. It's not necessarily a position for deep thrusting, so explore the pleasure to be had with her yoni being so tightly merged with his vajra. This is a good position for the woman to practice "milking" her man with her vaginal muscles. Also play with the excitement of subtle rocking movements as you imagine riding on the back of a huge, gentle beast.

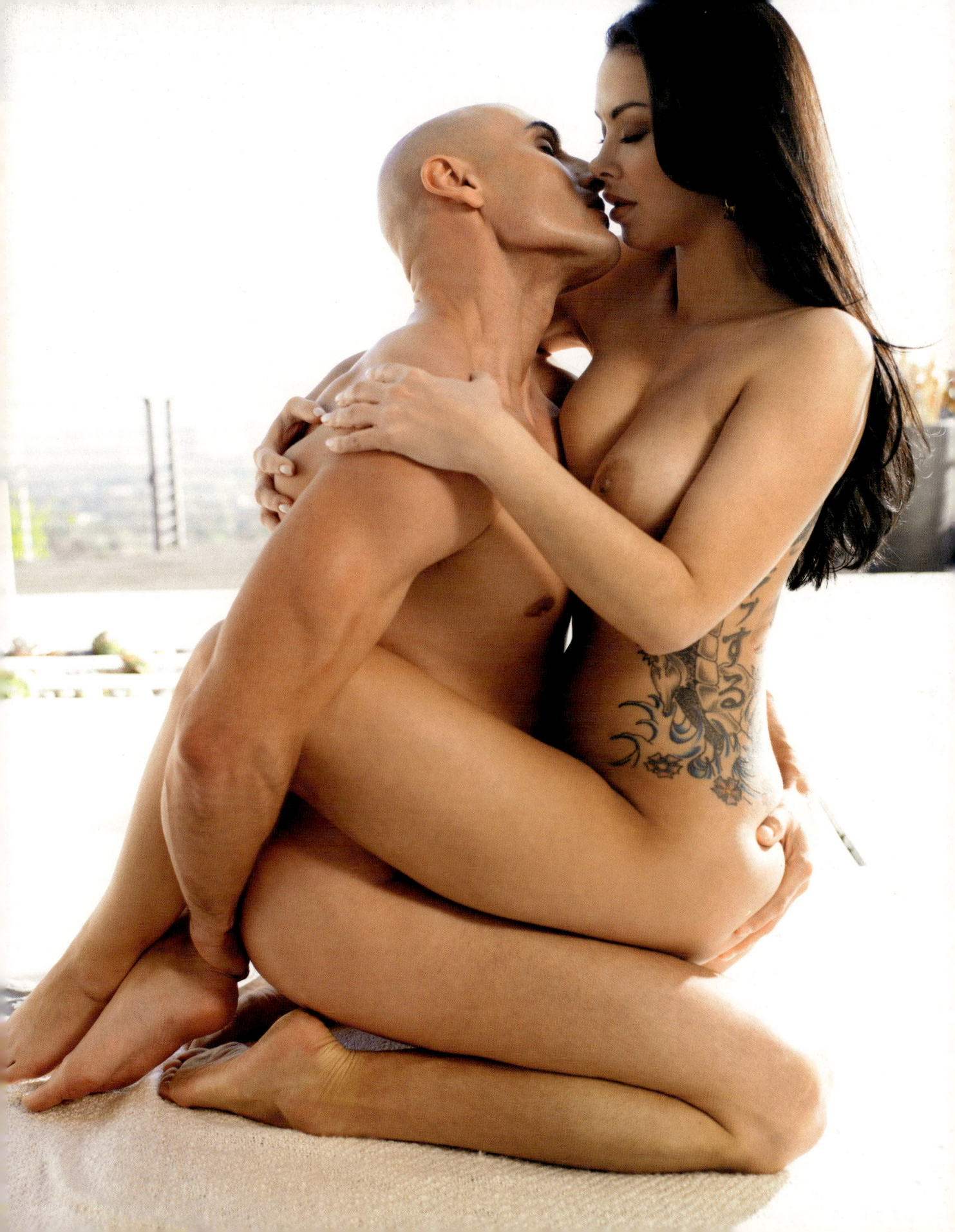

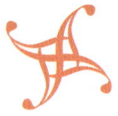

36 | THE PLOUGH

{ Turn Over Her Fertile Ground }

This posture offers the benefit of deep penetration for couples who want to try a more advanced pose. The final expression is visually beautiful, with the woman's legs stretched out powerfully behind her and the man kneeling forward into her. For many women, the feeling of complete surrender to the "driver" of the plough can be thrillingly erotic. Likewise, it can turn on the intensity of the sacred masculine, because men are in charge of all the movement in this position.

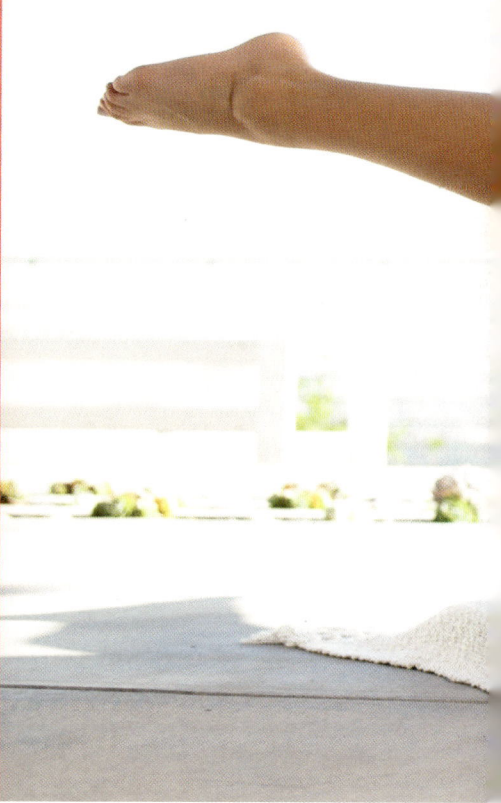

① Begin on a firm but well-padded surface. The man kneels with his knees together and invites his woman to sit on his lap facing away from him. She places her feet flat in front of her for balance. This is an ideal position to arouse one another. The man's arms are free to caress her breasts, belly, and legs. He can also kiss the back of her neck, breathe warmth into her hair, and whisper words of love or naughtiness into her ear. She can caress his legs, arch her back, and tease his vajra with her butt and stimulate her yoni as well.

② When you're sufficiently hot and bothered, the woman bends forward at the waist and reaches toward her feet in a prayer position. The man holds her around the waist and lifts her onto his erection.

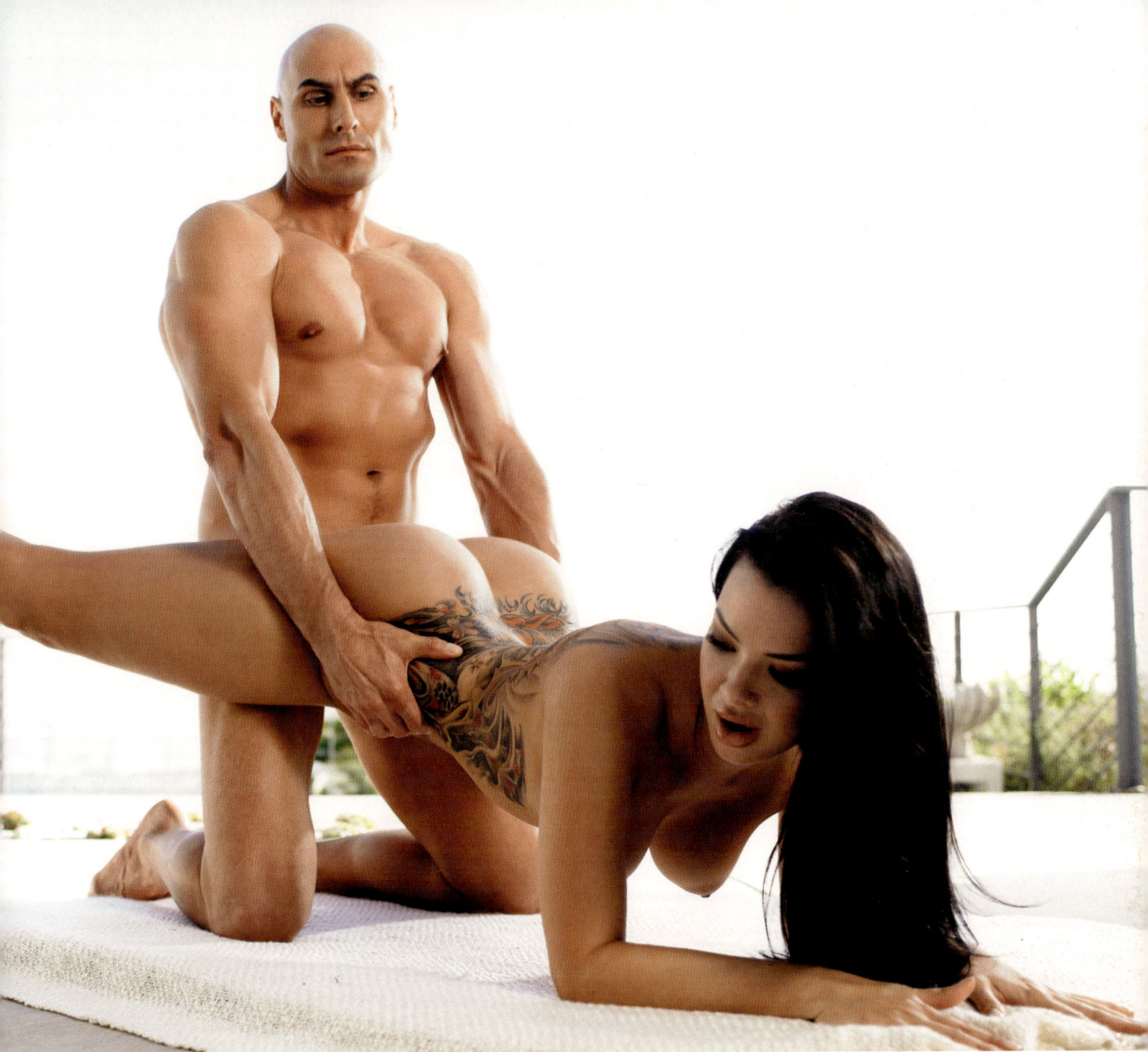

③ Placing her hands flat on the floor to support herself, she gently bends one leg and then the other alongside her man. He holds her firmly under the thighs as she straightens one leg at time back into a V shape behind him. She rests her weight on her forearms, which should be supported by a blanket or cushion for comfort. By pointing her toes, the woman can activate more grounding sexual energy by sending it out through her feet.

④ The man controls the movement by leaning forward and pulling her legs back as he drives into her. She can also match his rhythm by pressing into her forearms and rocking toward him as he moves into her. Enjoy unearthing a full harvest of sexual delights in this pose.

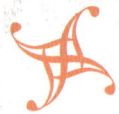

37 | OPEN FLOWER

❦ She Unfurls Her Petals in the Sun ❧

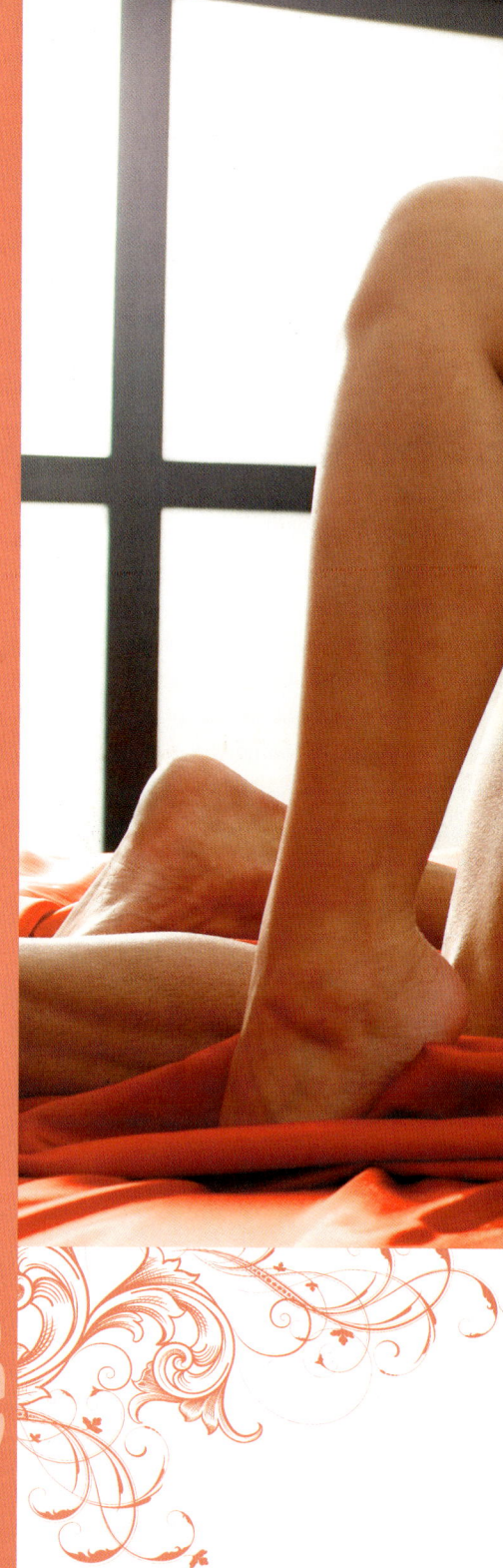

IN THIS MISSIONARY-POSITION VARIATION, the woman raises her pelvis up and opens her legs like a flower unfurling its petals in the sun. It is a fairly energetic pose in that the woman needs both upper-body and leg strength to support herself. It can be a powerful position for both men and women because the yoni is elevated for deeper penetration and the woman's legs are splayed open, making entry easy. Because the body is elevated higher than the head, this posture also stimulates the thyroid and the throat chakra of the woman, giving her courage to speak what is true.

"If we could recover a sense of the holiness of Eros and its creative, divine place in the nature of things, we might see how absurdly small our view of sex has been, and we might reinstate it without moralism at the center of life where it can offer vitality and intimacy of unrivaled power. Before we can give depth and richness to our sexuality, we have to discover the value of deep pleasure and desire and at the same time relax our anxious attention to the control of the emotions, the justification of our lives by work and restraint, and our belief in the value of repression and suffering."

—*Thomas Moore,* The Soul of Sex

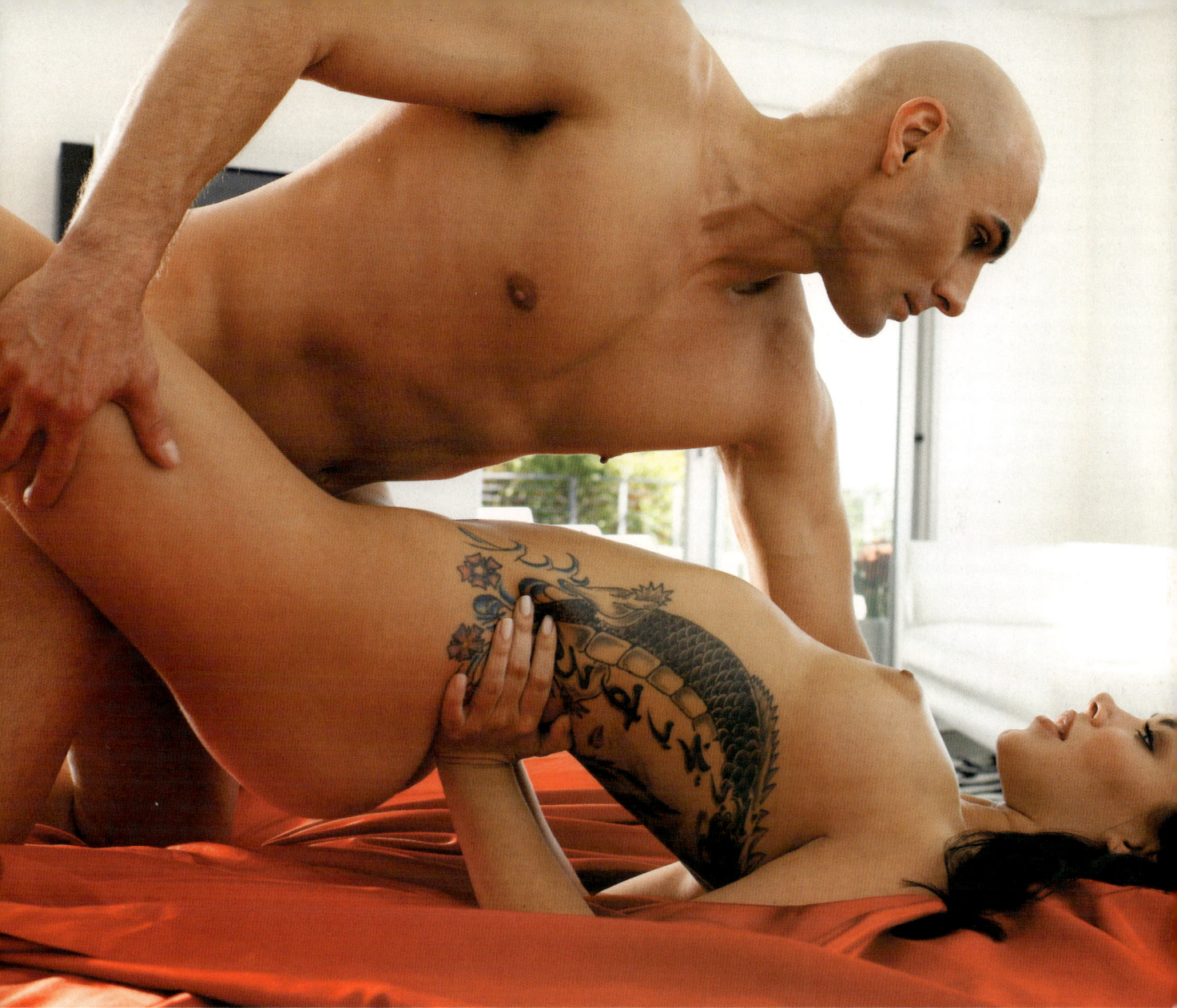

① The woman begins by getting herself into position, lying on her back and lifting her hips high off the bed. She comes up onto the balls of her feet and brings her feet as far back as is comfortable, ideally alongside or under her butt. She supports herself in this posture by drawing her shoulder blades back and together and placing her hands firmly underneath her hips.

② The man kneels between her legs, supporting his weight with his arms, and enters her open flower. He can also use one hand to fondle her breasts and stroke her face. Alternately, he can wrap one arm under her back to assist in supporting her weight and to facilitate deeper penetration.

38 | WHITE TIGER

{ Entice Him to Pounce }

THIS IS ANOTHER SEDUCTIVE rear-entry position where the woman entices the tiger in her man to pounce. Rear-entry postures can be highly erotic for both men and women. For the man, seeing the round curves of a woman's rear tends to be very provocative. For the woman, the postures often result in direct stimulation of her sacred spot. You'll both enjoy the deep penetration possible in this pose.

① The woman begins alone on the bed while the man stands back and enjoys watching her. Ladies, this is an opportunity to be playful. Consider starting off with a bit of clothing or lingerie and eventually pulling it to the side slowly to tease him with the sight and scent of you. If it doesn't interfere with lovemaking, it can be very sexy to leave it on partway or rip it off later. (Relatively inexpensive fishnet body stockings are easy to tear. Guys, discuss it with her beforehand, because shredding her favorite lingerie could unleash a different kind of tiger.)

② Women, think "feline" as you crawl slowly on the bed. Look over your shoulder frequently with your smoldering cat eyes and try some growls and purrs. Rotate your butt in the air and rock it back at him to simulate him thrusting inside you.

③ Men, wait as long as you can in order to build up the delicious anticipation, but eventually the tiger has to pounce! Women, keep one knee bent slightly and position several pillows under your hips and stomach. Although it's difficult to reach your clitoris in this position, rubbing yourself against the pillows is a great alternative to bring you to orgasm.

④ The man can rest his weight on outstretched arms or grab her around the waist. He can also pull her hair to tilt her head back, creating a deeper arch to her back as he thrusts passionately into her curves. Because this position can be very stimulating for the man, alternate slow and shallow thrusting with deeper, faster movements so that you both can enjoy lasting pleasure.

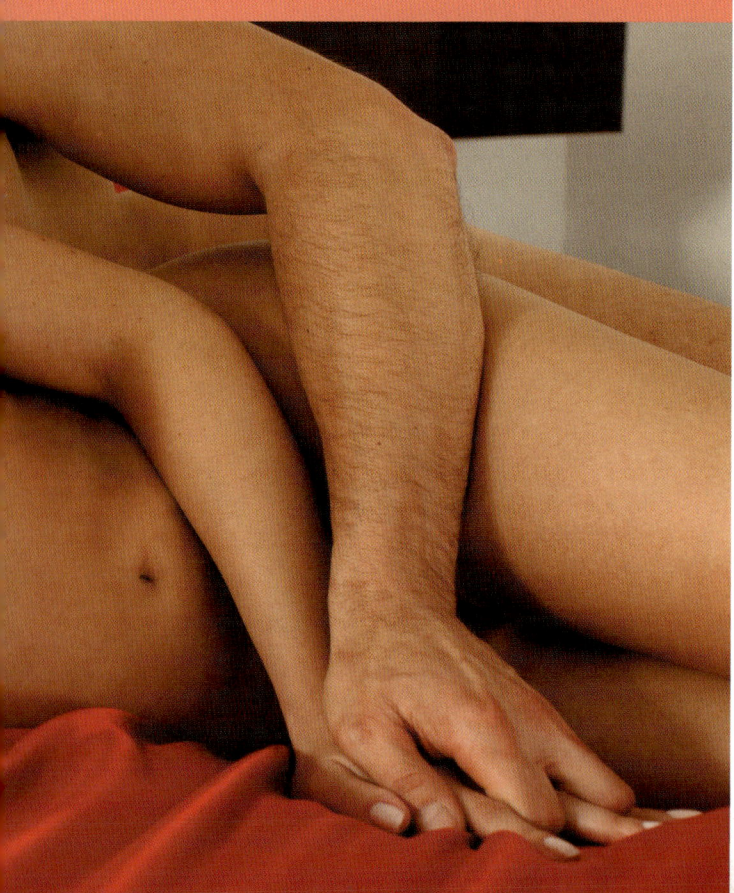

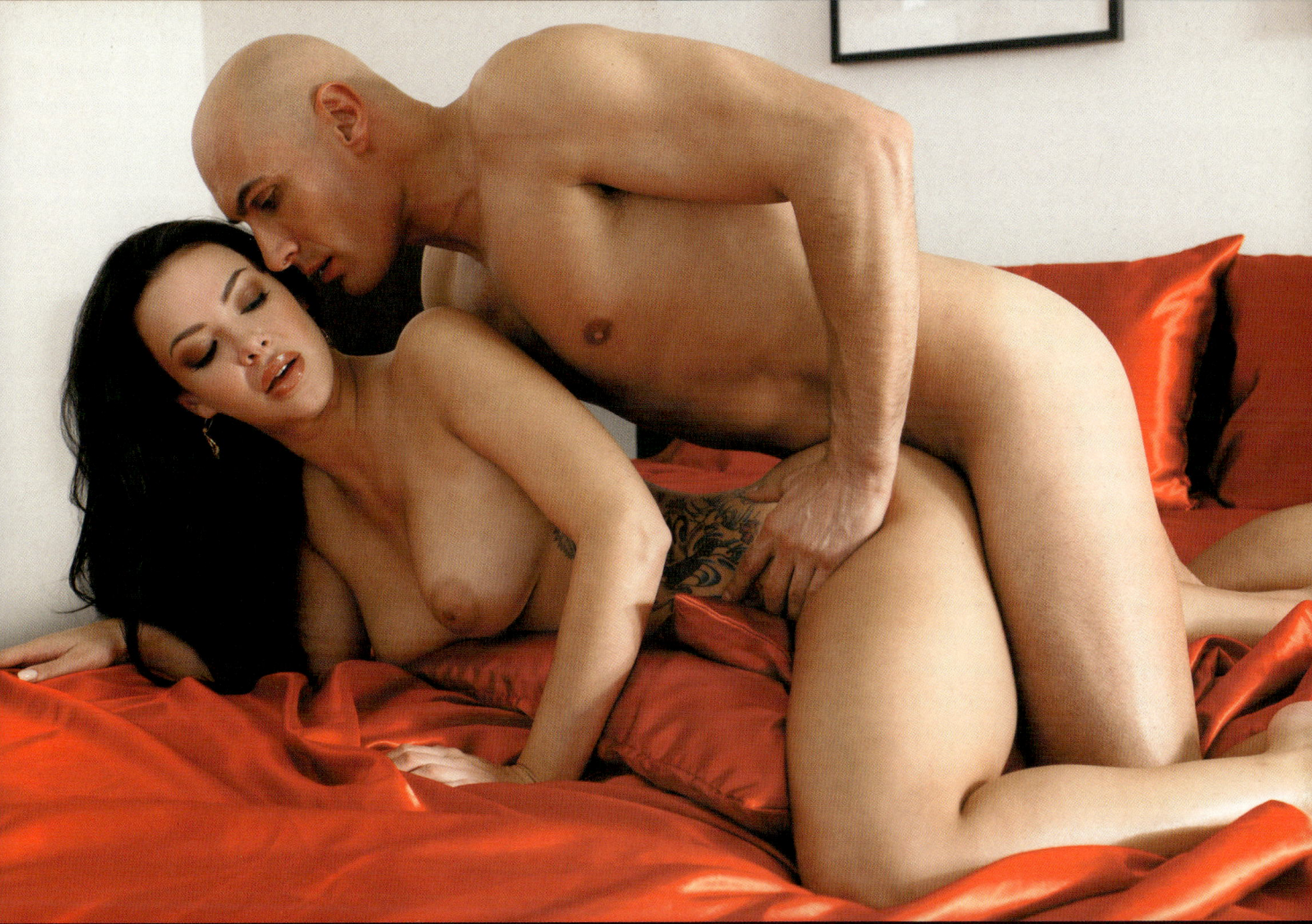

Make Some Noise

Sound is one of the three keys to moving sexual energy (the other two are breath and movement). Tap into your primal animal energy and vocalize during lovemaking. Although you might feel self-conscious at first, it's likely that your partner will get turned on hearing you growl, purr, or grunt like a beast.

You may be surprised at how sexually powerful you feel when you let yourself go. Vocalizing is one of the primary ways of increasing and expanding sexual energy by drawing it out of the pelvis and into the throat. Give each other permission to explore the deeper sexual responsiveness possible when you make bigger sounds.

Worried about the kids or the neighbors hearing? Let go and make no apologies. The Kama Sutra holds sexuality as an integrated part of life; the sounds of lovemaking are a joyful part of the symphony and are meant to be celebrated, not hushed.

39 | MOUNTAIN AND VALLEY

{ Meet in the Middle }

KAMA SUTRA TEACHINGS understand the dynamic interplay between opposites as a source of pleasure and passion: masculine and feminine, hard and soft, fast and slow, full and empty. Playful lovers explore both the mountains and the valleys in their lovemaking, honoring the view from the summit as well as the fertility of the land below. This pose sends healing energy into the womb and throat of the woman while the man taps into his sacred masculine strength. It is also a pose that promotes conception (so use it wisely).

This position requires some firm pillows or large bolsters. Ideally, the woman's hips should be raised high enough so that they are in alignment with her man when he's on his knees. His knees should be comfortably padded as well. This way, they can both relax into the pleasure of the pose without having to focus on support.

① Situate the woman on her back with her hips raised to meet her man's pelvis. To begin, he kneels between her legs and she relaxes her knees to the side and rests her feet on his calves. He can caress her legs and yoni or watch her play with herself as she gazes up at the rising mountain of her man. When you are both ready for penetration, he enters her.

② She raises one leg up to rest it on his shoulder and reaches out with the same hand to hold his. By holding hands, you can gently push and pull together, finding your rhythm. This is an ideal position for the man to practice a series of shallow thrusts (try seven) followed by one long, slow, and deep thrust. This should be a comfortable position for both of you. When the woman's leg tires, switch to the other one. Notice the variations in the angle of penetration and how that feels to both of you. Maintain eye contact up to and through your orgasmic peak.

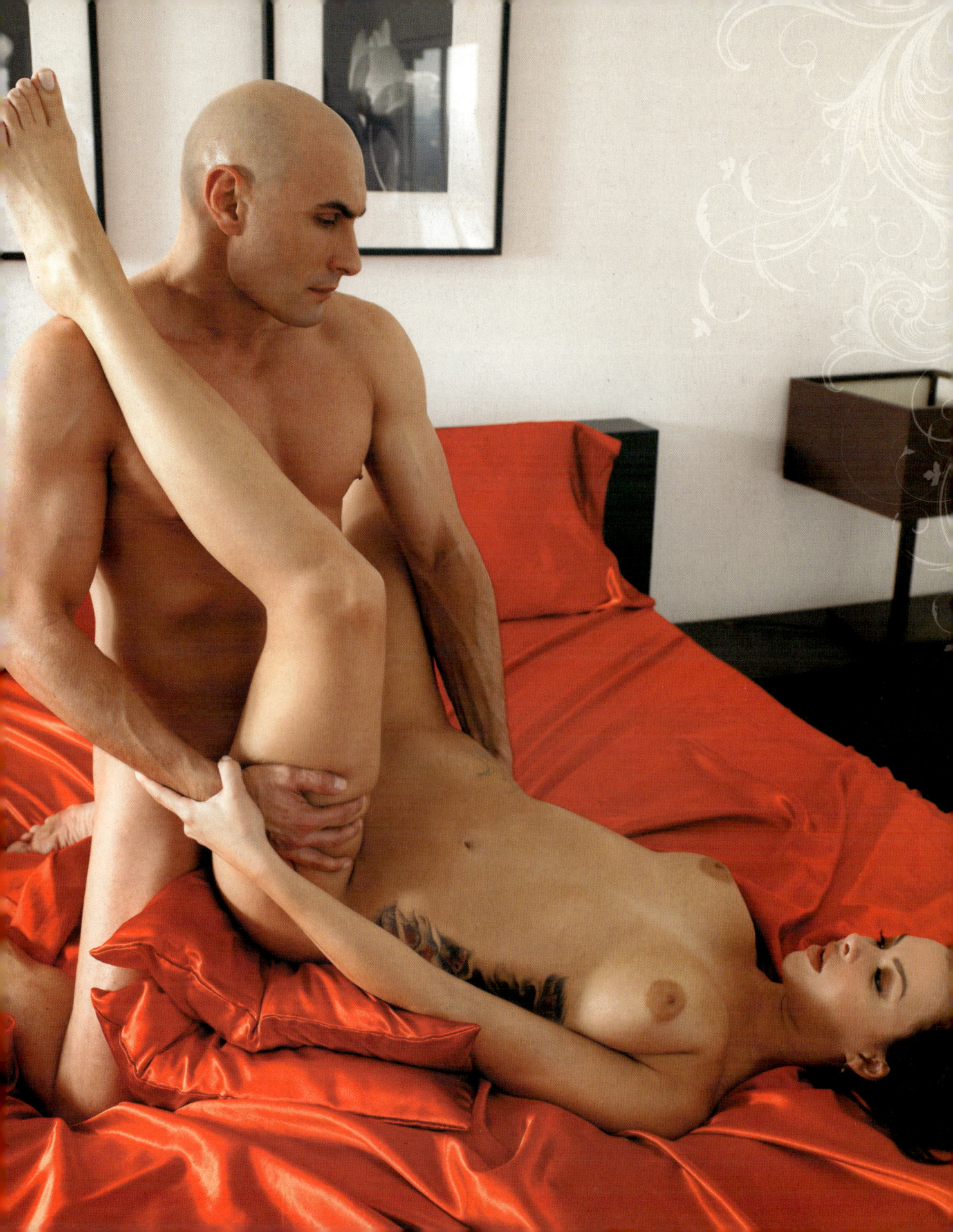

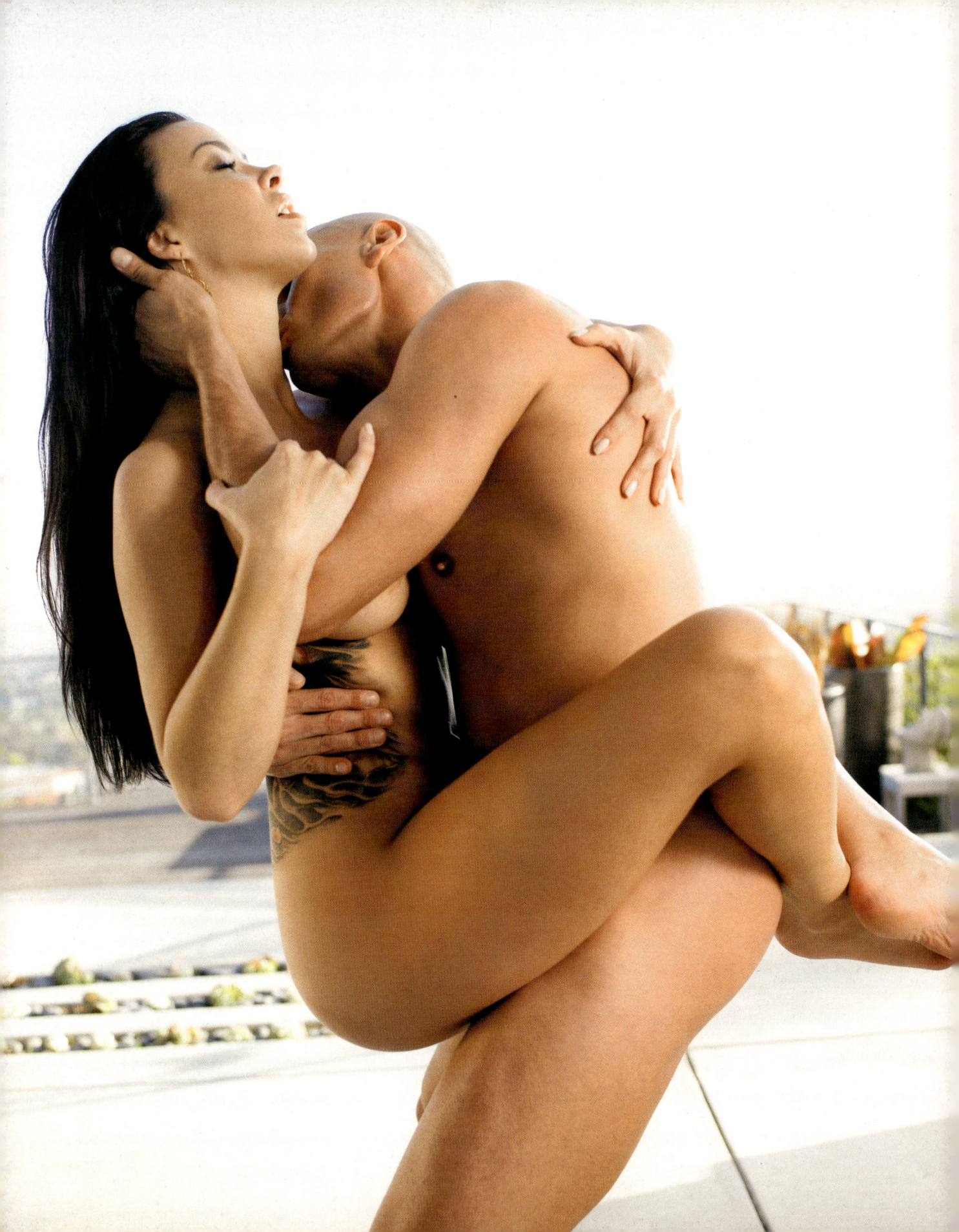

Magnetic Attraction

Vatsyayana made note of the differences between men and women in terms of their sex drive and their anatomical dimensions. He had three categories for the level of "carnal desire or force of passion" that a man or woman possessed as "small, middling, or intense." Depending on "the depth of her yoni," a woman was a "deer, mare, or elephant." Men were categorized according to the size of their vajra as a "hare, bull, or horse." All these factors made for combinations of "high and low unions," with the best partners being those who matched up or were adjacent in terms of their size and desire.

Although these ideas offer some practical perspective, there's no need for today's Kama Sutra lovers to get locked into any restrictive categories. Explore the Kama Sutra positions to find the ones that give you and your lover the most pleasure, and expect that to evolve. In terms of the level of passion you have together, keep in mind the wisdom of the magnet. The more distinct the two poles, the more intense the attraction. Poles that are the same repel, not attract.

For example, if you are a high-powered professional woman in the outside world who longs for a "real" man in the bedroom who will press you up against a wall, pull off your clothes, throw you down, and take you, then don't act like a man by ordering him around and telling him what to do (although it's fine to share your fantasy with him ahead of time). To call forth his masculine energy, drop fully into your feminine energy by accessing your softness, vulnerability, openness, and juicy sensuality.

Although most women at their core are feminine and most men are masculine, it doesn't matter who takes on which pole (indeed, adept lovers delight in switching up the roles). What is most important is not competing for the same pole or hanging out in the middle, which can make for a harmonious friendship but not a lot of passion in the bedroom.

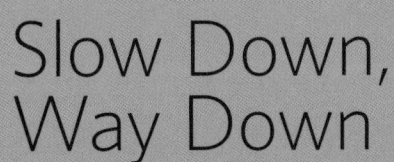

Slow Down, Way Down

The Kama Sutra elaborately describes courtship and seduction procedures, including how to woo a maiden, decipher her glances, and nurture her confidence. Days of foreplay are recommended before engaging in sex. Take your time, it warns, because "women being of a tender nature, want tender beginnings, and when they are forcibly approached by men . . . they sometimes suddenly become haters of sexual connection, and sometimes even haters of the male sex."

Vatsyayana further warns, "You ardent young men, don't forget foreplay! You are here to satisfy your woman. Listen to what she wants, to the way of her desire . . . neglect no smallest part of her body. The man should make it his duty to discover them, and once found to show his lover the refined pleasures to be had there."

The frenetic goal orientation in the West often has us so overly focused on racing to orgasm that we miss the ecstasy of the journey. The first step is to notice that you're thinking about the future and pushing toward orgasm. When you realize that you're "there" and not "here," relax and pay attention to where you feel pleasure in your body in this moment. Breathe into that place and see whether you can allow the pleasure to open and expand right here, right now. Slowing down will get you off the speeding highway so that you notice new avenues and alleyways that can guide you to delightful places you've never been before. Kama Sutra lovers don't want to rush to the end; they want to expand the pleasure as long as possible.

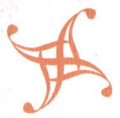

40 | A PANTHER SPRINGS

⟨ Take Her with Passion from Behind ⟩

WE LOVE THE MYSTERIOUS quality of a panther—the fierce intensity blended with feline grace. In the cat world, males commonly grab the fur on the back of the female's neck in their mouth as they mount her. Similarly, in this Kama Sutra position, the woman lies prone and undefended while her man takes her with passion from behind.

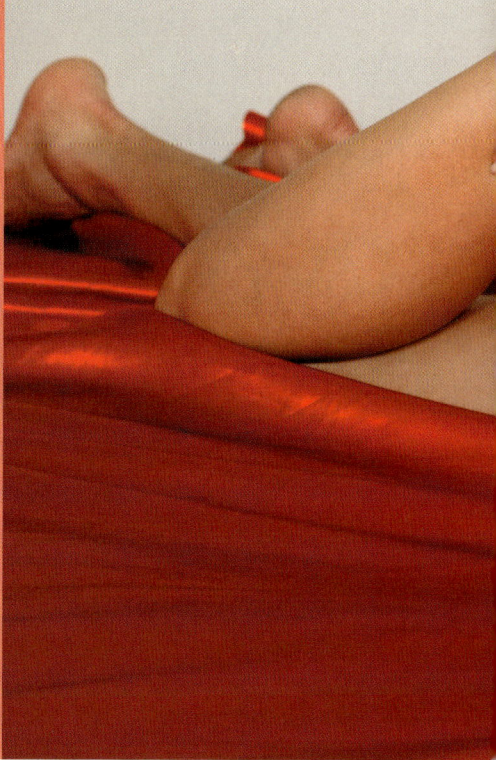

① The woman lies flat on her belly on a firm bed or surface (watch that her back doesn't sway too much). Place a pillow under her head and a thick quilt or blanket underneath her for padding. She then bends her knees backward and grasps her ankles firmly in her hands. This puts her in a gentle backbend position that opens the whole front of her body.

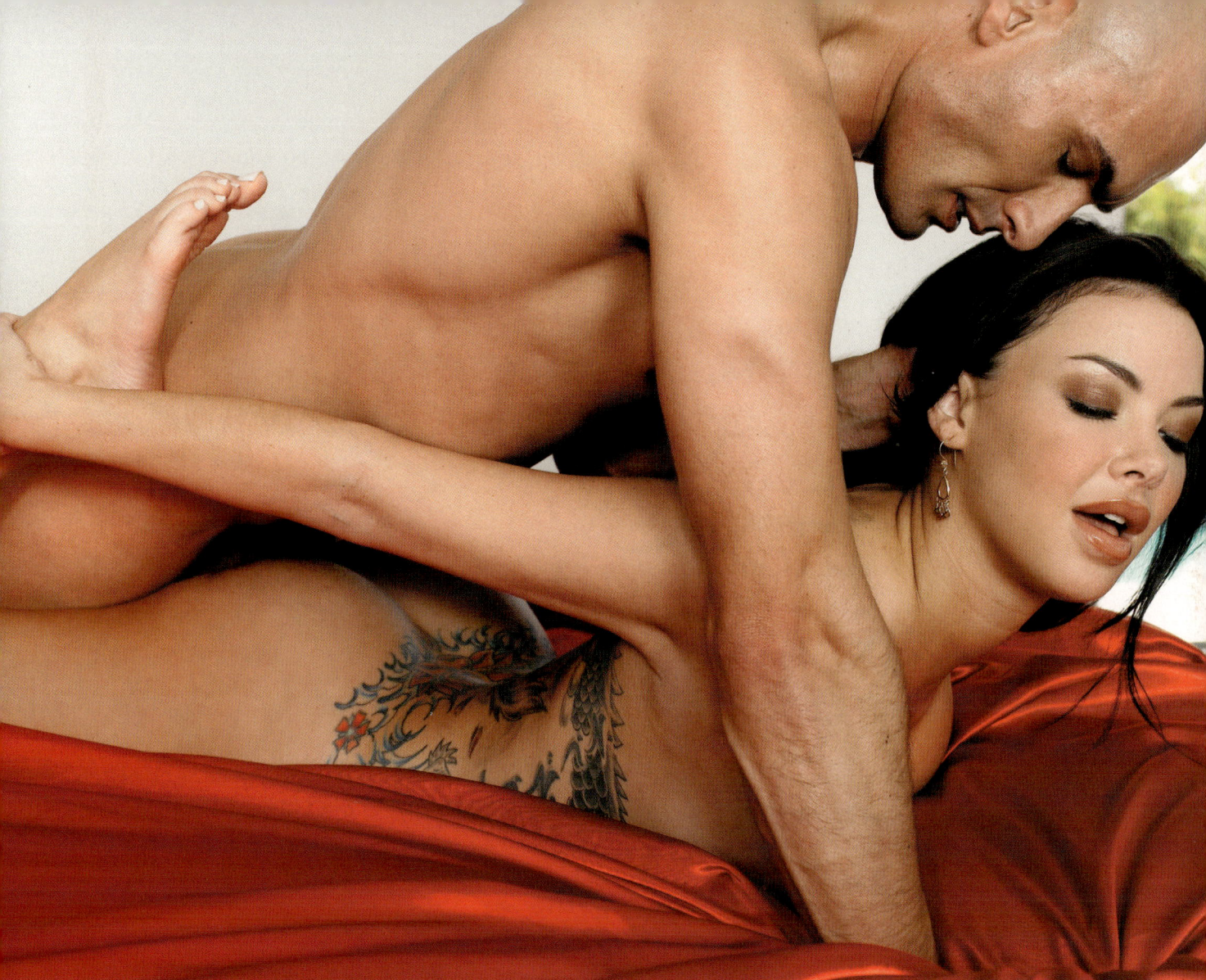

② He then approaches her from behind, kneeling between her thighs. Before entering her, he can arouse you both by gently gliding his vajra up and down the cleft of her butt, using a good lubricant. He then enters her and alternates shallow, slow thrusts with more vigorous, deep thrusting. Depending on the strength and flexibility of the woman, she can squeeze her legs more tightly together or open them more widely for a variety of sensations.

③ If you choose, the man can grab a handful of the woman's hair or bite and suck the back of her neck in an erotic role-play of the panther dominating his mate. He can also come down onto this elbows or slide his arm under her armpit to hold on to the front of her shoulder and pull her gently into a deeper backbend (stay in good communication and, of course, make adjustments to protect yourself from strain).

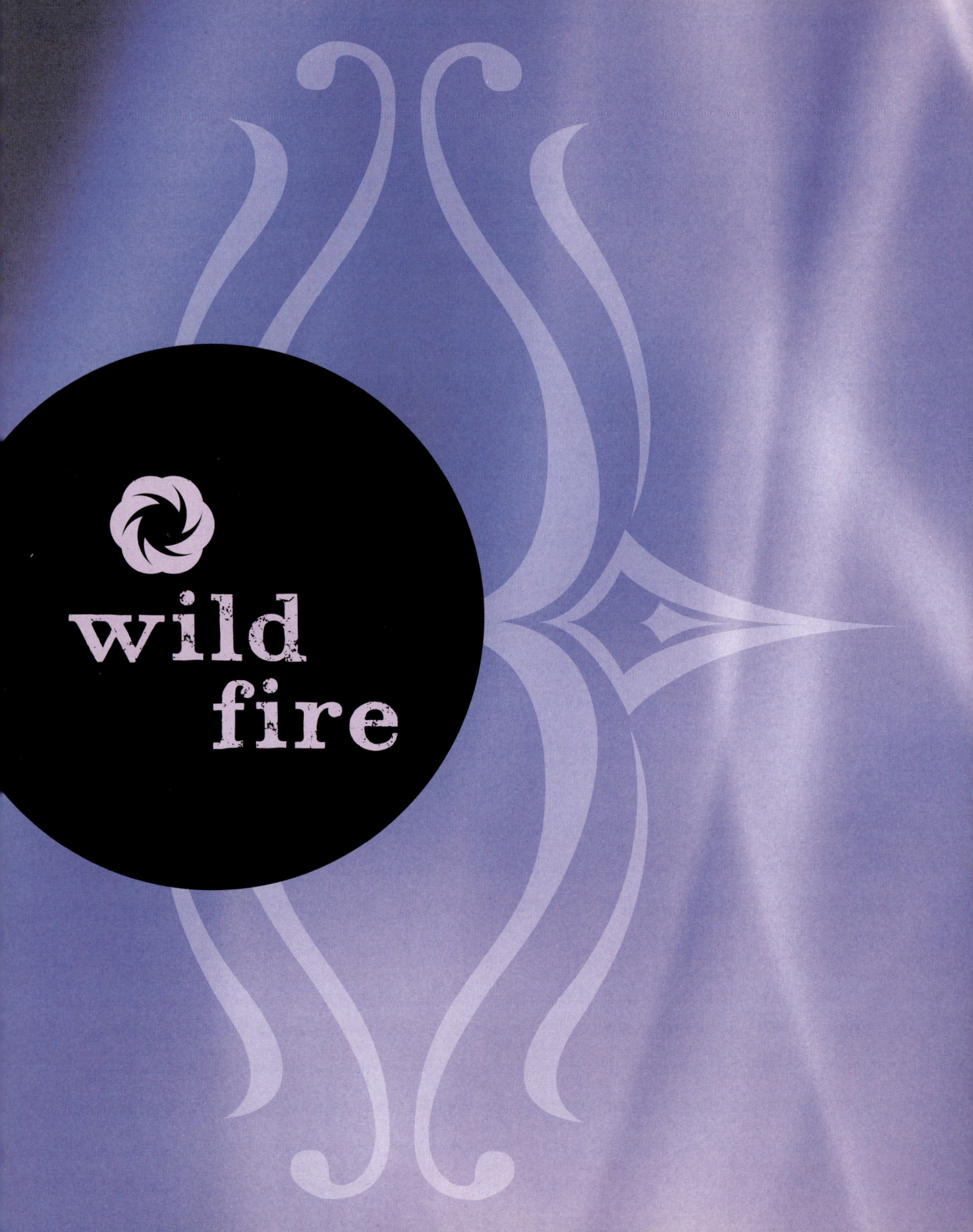

wild
fire

HOW HOT CAN YOU TAKE IT? SOMETIMES THE FIRE KNOWS NO BOUNDS AND THE INFERNO RAGES IN ALL DIRECTIONS. PASSION SWEEPS YOU OFF YOUR FEET AND YOU FEEL DELICIOUSLY LOST IN THE HEAT OF THIS TIMELESS MOMENT. TAKE A WALK ON THE WILD SIDE WITH THESE SCORCHING MOVES, BEST FOR THE MOST ATHLETIC AND ADVENTUROUS OF KAMA SUTRA LOVERS.

41 | THE FROG

{ Fast and Deep from the Haunches }

THE MAN NEEDS STRONG haunches in this position, just like a frog, so that his vajra can "leap" inside her yoni and bring you both to heights of pleasure. In this position of deep penetration, the woman remains relatively still outwardly, using her Love Pump (page 69) to pleasure you both. The beginning stages offer the opportunity for intimate embracing, allowing the woman to surrender into being totally held by her lover.

① Start on a firm surface, ideally with adequate cushions set up for the woman to lie back in comfortably for the final position with her hips raised high. The man squats down with his feet flat on the floor and his knees open wide. You can also try this position with the man's back against a wall to give him greater support.

② The woman sits on his lap, embraces him, and either keeps her feet on the floor behind him or braces them against the wall for balance and to support some of her weight. When you're both ready, the woman guides his vajra inside her. He can rock her gently or bounce her up and down using his haunches. Alternatively, he can remain still while she flexes her Love Pump to bring you both pleasure.

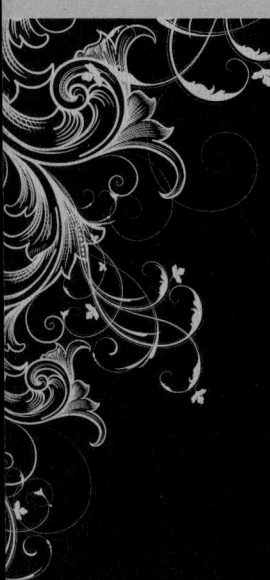

Leaving Your Mark

The Kama Sutra goes into elaborate detail about marking and biting your partner, which happens between "those that are intensely passionate" and "to whom the practice is agreeable." Vatsyayana describes exactly how to create various marks with the fingernails, including "tiger claw, peacock's foot, half moon and circle, blue lotus, and jump of a hare," to mention but a few of the ways one can leave a "token of remembrance" on a lover. He says that noticing the emblem of passion proudly displayed on a woman's breast or a man's neck is likely to spark "love and respect" in others.

Although modern readers may find these ancient practices distasteful or abusive, passionate lovers know about the delicate dance between pleasure and pain. In the heat of the moment, a little pain can catapult you up to a new level of excitement and sensation.

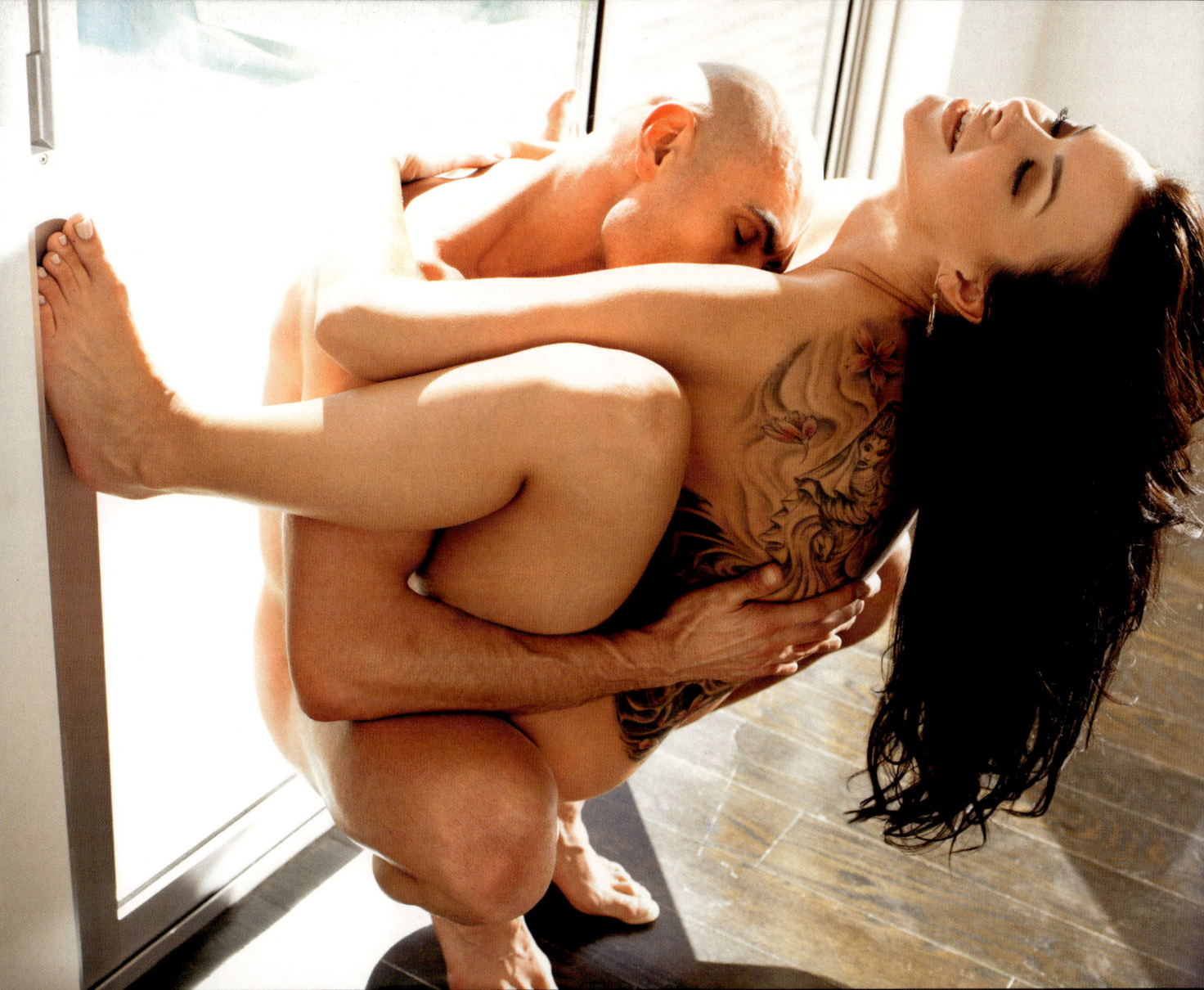

Talk to your partner about your desires ahead of time. If you want to get really edgy and play with bondage/discipline, dominance/submission, or sadomasochism (commonly referred to as BDSM), make sure it's consensual. Then have a "safe word" that you can use to stop everything immediately if you need to, a code word you wouldn't normally use in the bedroom, such as "magenta" or "daisy." Don't use common words like "no" or "stop" because those might be words that you want to use when role-playing (as in "No—Stop— you dirty old pirate!").

42 | SHIVA'S DANCE

{ *A Standing Celebration of the Powerful Masculine* }

A NATURAL TRANSITION from The Frog, this position is a passionate celebration of the god Shiva, worshiped throughout India as the embodiment of sacred masculine power, in ecstatic embrace with his goddess Shakti. In this high-energy position, they join in a sacred dance together as Shakti throws her legs around Shiva while he stands fully erect. Called "Supported Congress" in the Kama Sutra, this standing posture is good for fast, energetic sex and will require some stamina for both of you.

① If you're not moving to this position from The Frog, begin with the woman sitting on the edge of a bed or chair with her knees wide open. The man squats low in front of her so she can wrap her legs around him. He enters her from this position. She wraps her arms around his shoulders and neck, pressing down (rather than pulling his neck forward) to support her weight. She also buoys herself by using her inner thigh muscles to squeeze him around the waist as she clasps her feet tightly behind him.

② He comes to a standing position, holding her either around her waist or under her butt as he presses into her. By using her upper-body and leg strength, she can gyrate and rock against him as well.

③ When one or both of you fatigue, the man squats down again or slowly lowers the woman back to a seated position on the edge of the bed while staying inside her, if possible. This is the ideal moment to maintain deep eye contact, breathe, circulate sexual energy, and use the stillness to build up orgasmic potential.

④ When your bodies want to move together again, the woman wraps her legs tightly around the man and he lifts her up again. In this way, you can cycle through several rounds of this posture and build to a powerful climax.

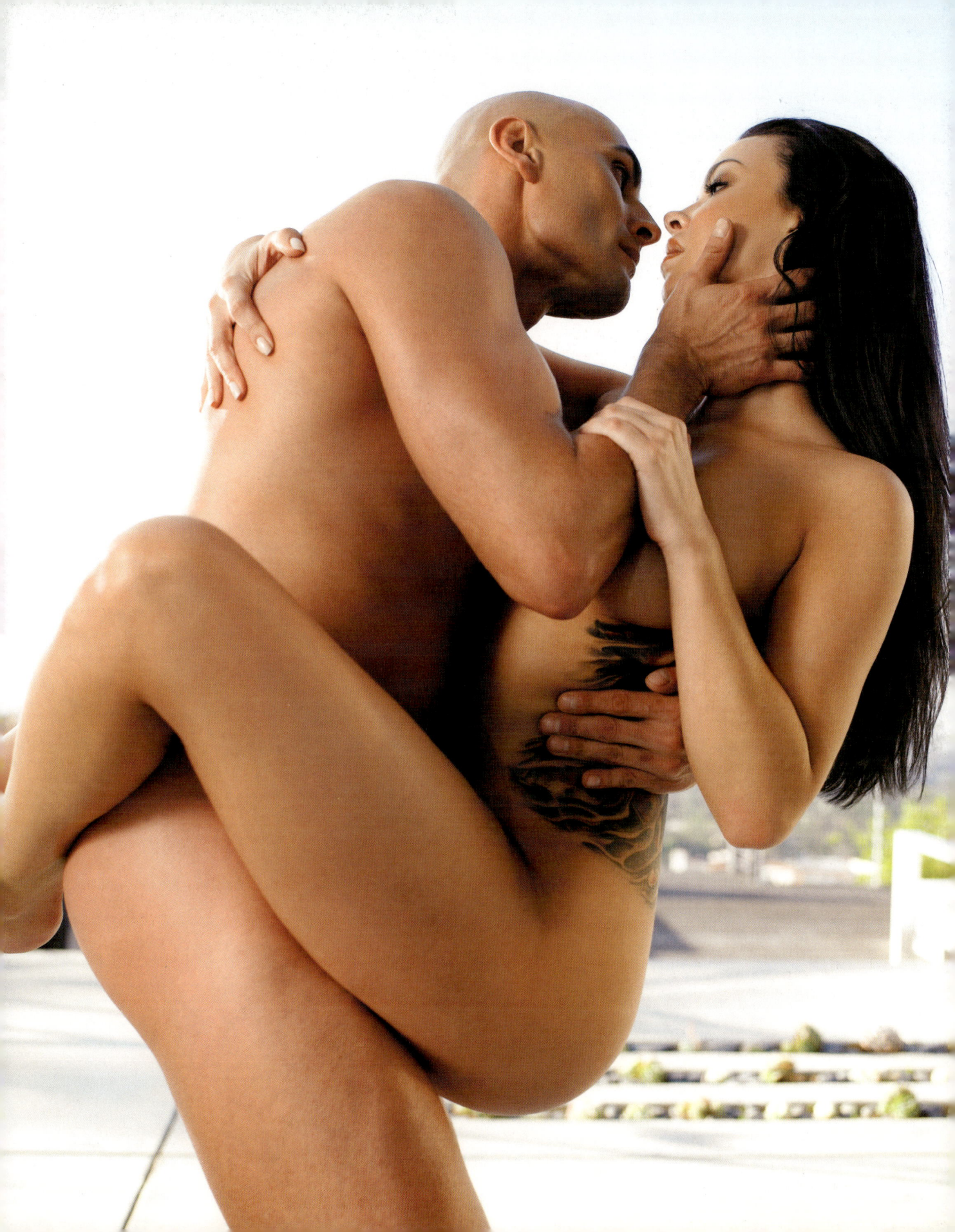

43 | BUTTERFLY

[A Balancing Flight to Ecstasy]

ALTHOUGH THE RANGE of motion is limited in this strenuous balancing posture, the intensity of it can be exciting because the woman is suspended by her man and opens her wings like a butterfly. The man needs good upper-body strength to support the weight of the woman, and care must be taken to not strain his neck or back. Make sure in the heat of passion that you stay in communication if anything begins to hurt. It may also be best to try this position on a firm surface so that the man has traction for balance.

① The man kneels with his knees together and sits back on his feet. The woman sits on his lap, wrapping her feet around him. Here you can enjoy embracing and caressing as you build passion and prepare for intercourse.

② The man raises his left knee so that it is at a right angle to his body. As he does this, the woman balances herself by holding firmly around his neck and standing up slightly on her feet to assist him in entering her. Once he is inside her, she leans into his bent knee as he holds her around the lower back.

③ She then lifts her left leg up over his right arm resting it in his elbow crease. She raises her right leg up to rest on his left shoulder which will fully open her butterfly wings. He cradles her while she leans back, holding him around the neck. Alternatively, she can keep her right leg down and use her leverage to press into him. The woman should focus on pressing down on his shoulders rather than pulling forward on his neck as she rocks toward him.

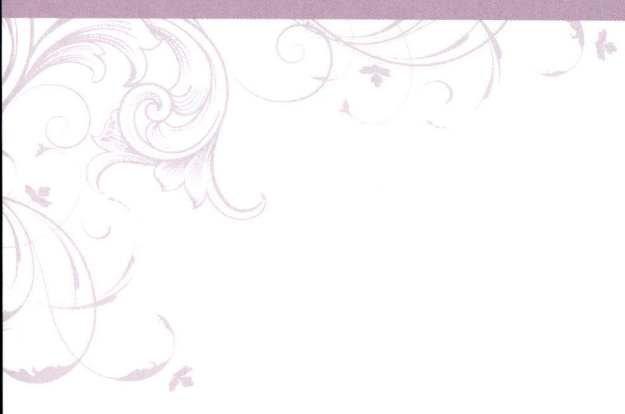

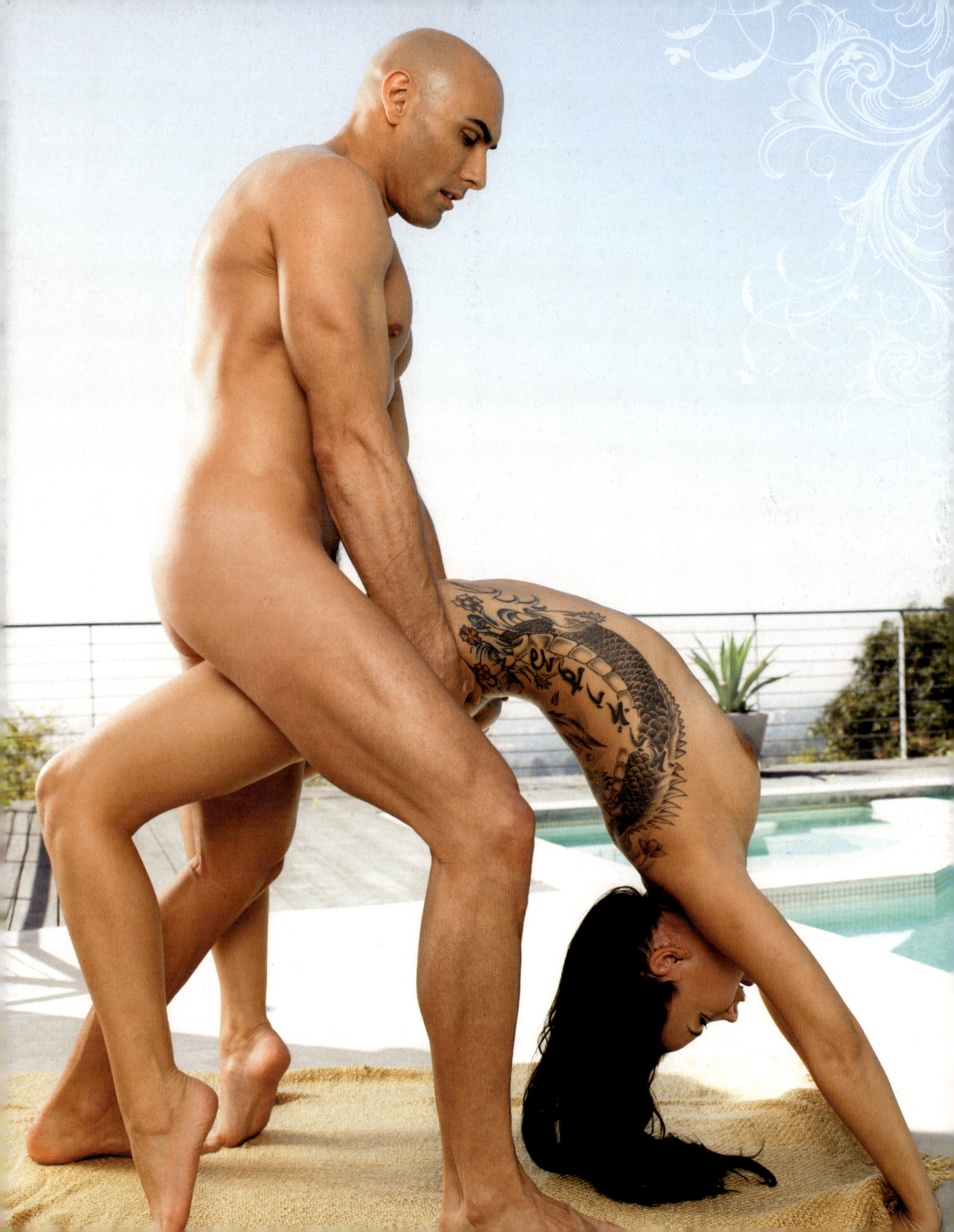

46 | THE HUNTER

{ Falling Prey to Ecstasy }

THIS POSE ALLOWS A MAN to access his inner warrior as he captures his woman in a passionate embrace. If he is able to do so with confidence, the woman will be able to surrender to him completely. Many women long to be taken by the power of the sacred masculine and his "arrow" of focused intent. Although it may be the hunter who sweeps her off her feet, the posture is most exciting when the woman takes control of sexually stimulating them both by flexing her Love Pump (page 69).

① Begin by facing each other on a firm but padded surface so that the man's knee will be protected while bearing weight in the pose. The man kneels down on his right knee with his left leg out at a right angle to his body, grasping the woman around her waist. The woman nestles her right foot on his left hip bone crease and places her hands on his shoulders, keeping her standing leg straight.

② When she's ready, she slowly bends her right leg and lowers herself to sit on his left leg. Her right foot will naturally slide around to his lower back as she uses it to pull herself closer to him. Her left arm circles around his neck. Hold and caress each other, feeling your genitals pressed together.

③ As the passion builds, he circles his arm firmly around her lower back, tilts her backward so that she must hang on to him for balance, and enters her in that moment of vulnerability. By engaging his abdominal muscles and using the strength of his upper body, he can hold her without straining his back. She can assist him by using her upper-body strength to press down on his shoulders, never straining his neck.

④ Then she tightens her right leg around his body to hold him close while she drops her left knee down and grasps the top of her left foot with her left hand. This brings her into a more upright position. As she pumps her yoni and internally squeezes his vajra, she arches back and lets her head go in erotic surrender.

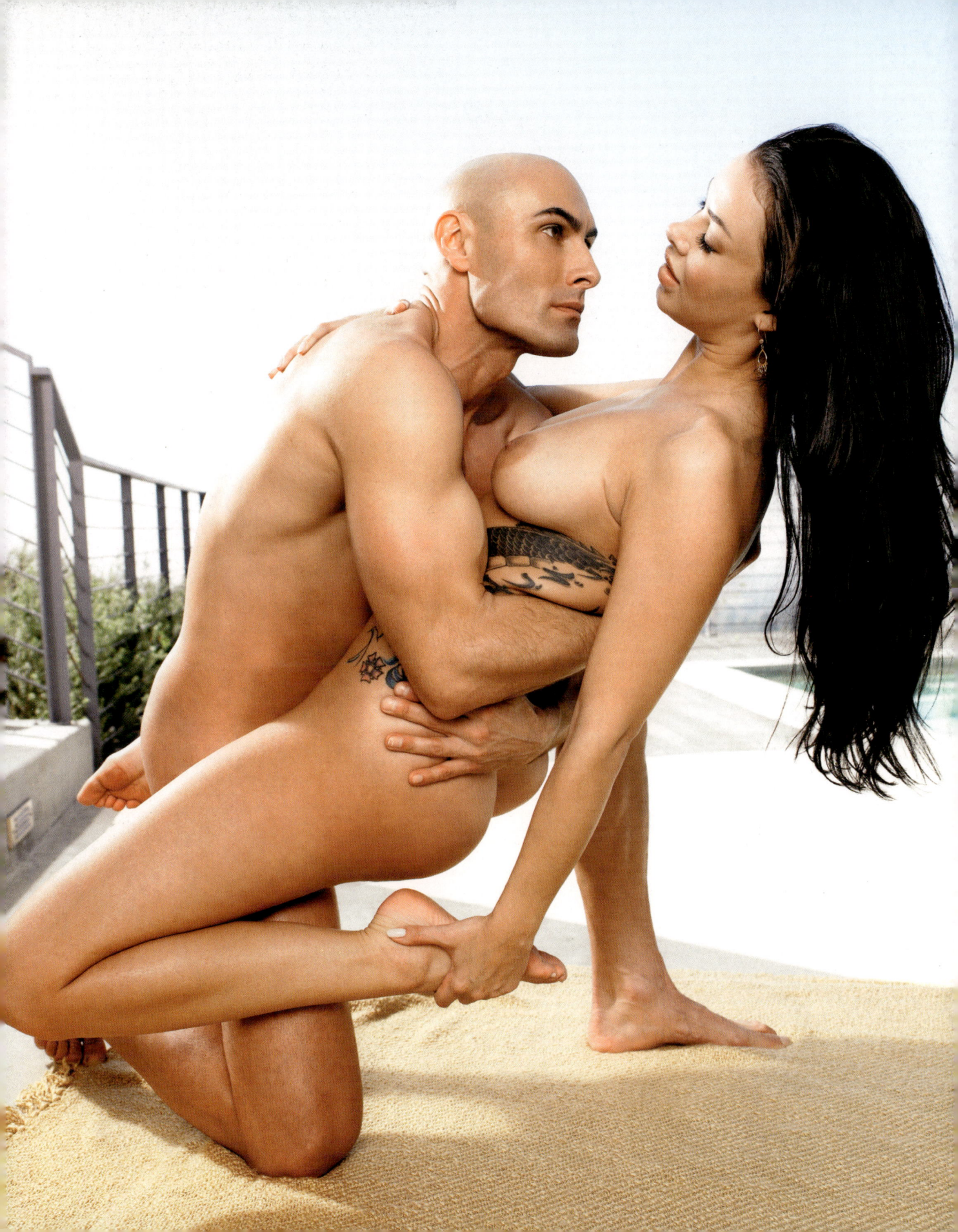

47 | THE SERPENT

{ Surrender to Upside-Down Temptation }

IN THIS, ONE OF THE MOST difficult of the Kama Sutra postures, a woman must have a strong upper body and a very flexible back. The man must be *certain* that he has the strength to hold her while she's upside down. Although the final expression of the pose offers limited movement and penetration may be shallow, the sheer athleticism of the posture, which requires a blend of grace and balance, can be liberating.

① The woman begins by standing in front of her man with her back to him. She inhales and brings her arms up, touches her hands over her head, and then exhales, swan diving into a standing forward bend, placing her palms flat on the floor. The man moves close to her and nuzzles her from behind, fondling her hips, back, and butt.

② The man secures solid footing and slightly bends his right leg forward to anchor himself. The woman raises her right leg so that her knee is bent and the top of her foot presses against his right armpit. When she has her balance on one leg, she brings her left foot up as well. Now she is supporting her weight in a handstand. She also presses the tops of her feet into his shoulders as she arches her back and opens herself to him. The man enters her, holding on to her thighs firmly to support her.

③ In the final stage of the pose, the man lowers her down to a large, firm bolster pillow (set under a blanket, if desired) as she bends her arms. She turns her head and comes to rest with her cheek and shoulder on the bolster. She continues to support some of her weight with her arms and, depending on the height of the bolster, may rest on her forearms as well. She can also grab his ankle with the hand closest to his feet and use that grip as leverage for pressing her yoni into her man. Her cervical spine can be prone to injury in this posture so the man must be certain he can hold her firmly without any undue pressure on her neck. For a break, or for more vigorous lovemaking, the couple can return to step 2 of the posture.

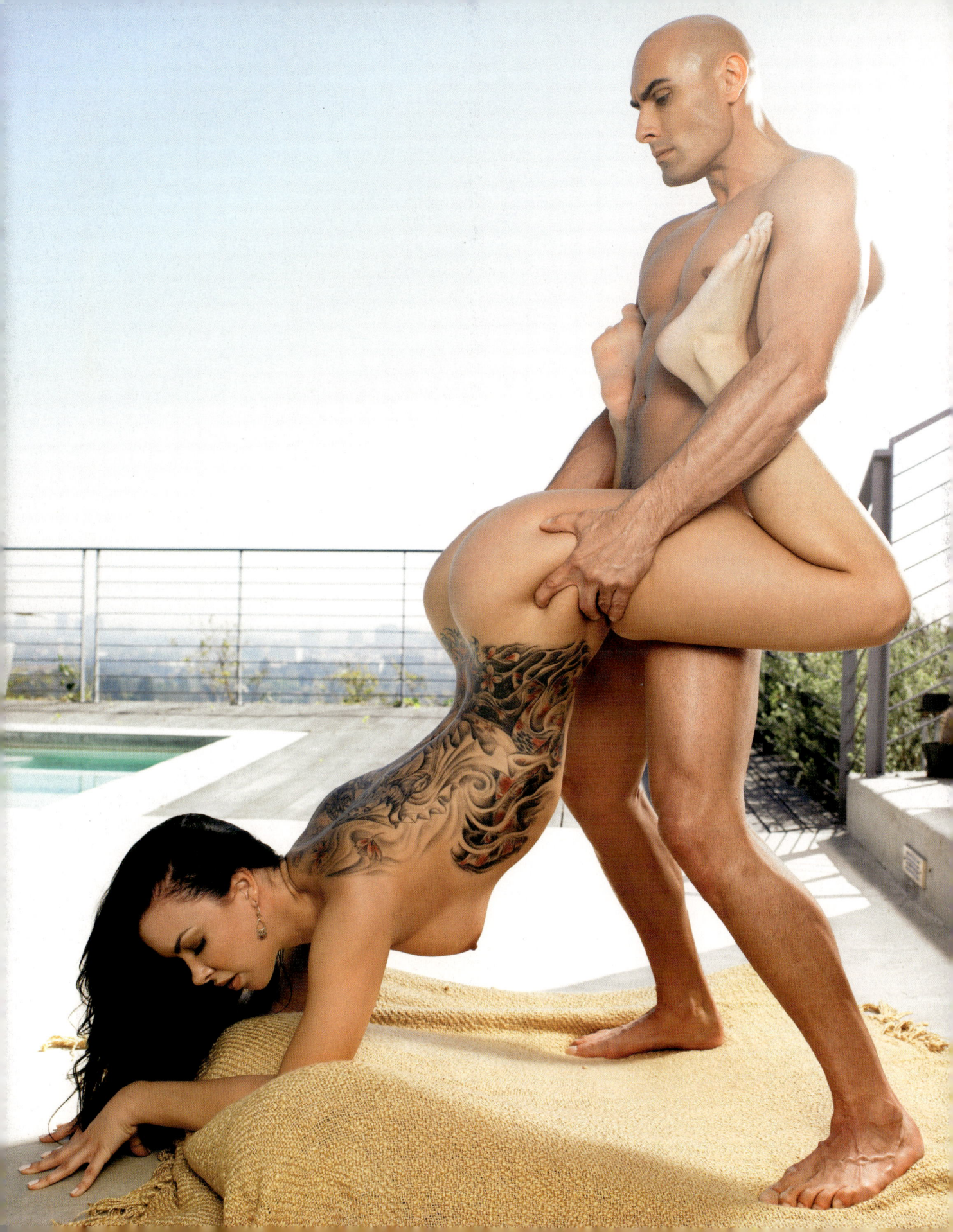

48 | SPINNING TOP

{ Front to Back and Begging for More }

VATSYAYANA RECOMMENDS this classic, although advanced, Kama Sutra posture as another alternative for the sexually energetic woman who may be with a fatigued or lower libido man. And men don't have to fit into either category to be turned on by this steamy position that offers a very sexy view of their woman. It has the added benefit of being a perfect posture to anally stimulate your woman or massage her butt. Ideally, this position is done on a bench so that in the final expression the woman can fully straddle her man and press into the floor with her feet for leverage.

① The man lies down on his back with comfortable padding and pillows underneath him, his knees apart and bent slightly. The woman straddles him, taking him inside her, with her knees alongside his body and her feet hooking underneath his thighs. She places her hands on the bench behind her, inside his knees, with her palms flat; she arches back, letting her head and neck go. The man can hold on to her hips to help support her in the backbend as she opens her heart and yoni to him.

② The woman straightens her legs out so that her feet are alongside his head. She then carefully lifts one leg over his head to join the other. Then, supporting herself and being careful not to twist his vajra, she slowly "spins" around so that she is still sitting on him but facing away from him with her legs and feet now inside his open legs.

③ She lowers her legs down to the ground on either side of him, straddling him again but in the opposite direction. If the man is practiced in yoga and has a strong back, he can arch up so that the middle of his back is raised, which may lift the woman higher for a different angle of penetration. If not, she can use her leg muscles to press into the ground, rocking back and forth to stimulate them both. Alternatively, the woman can rest her knees alongside him on the bench if she cannot reach the ground or wants to try a different angle.

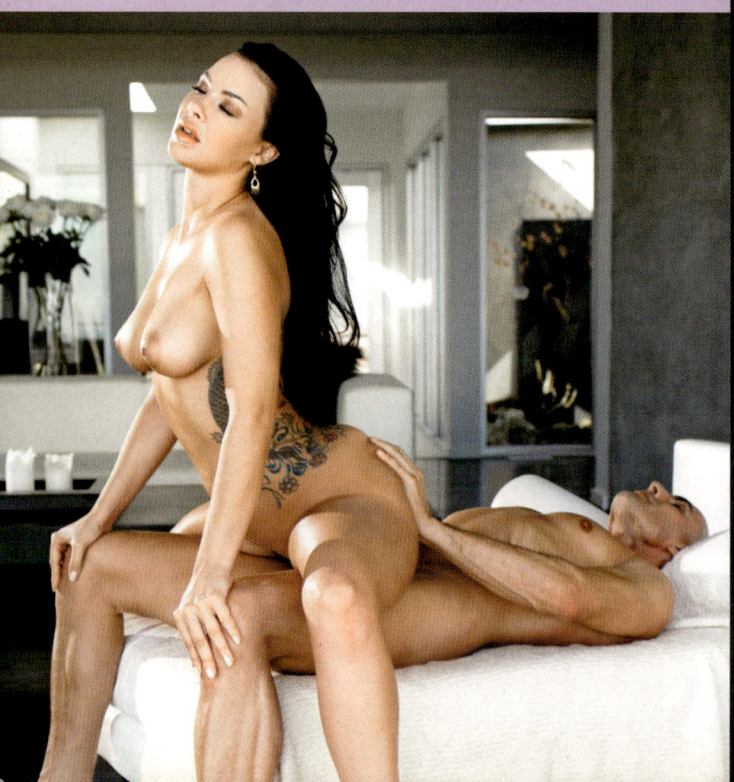

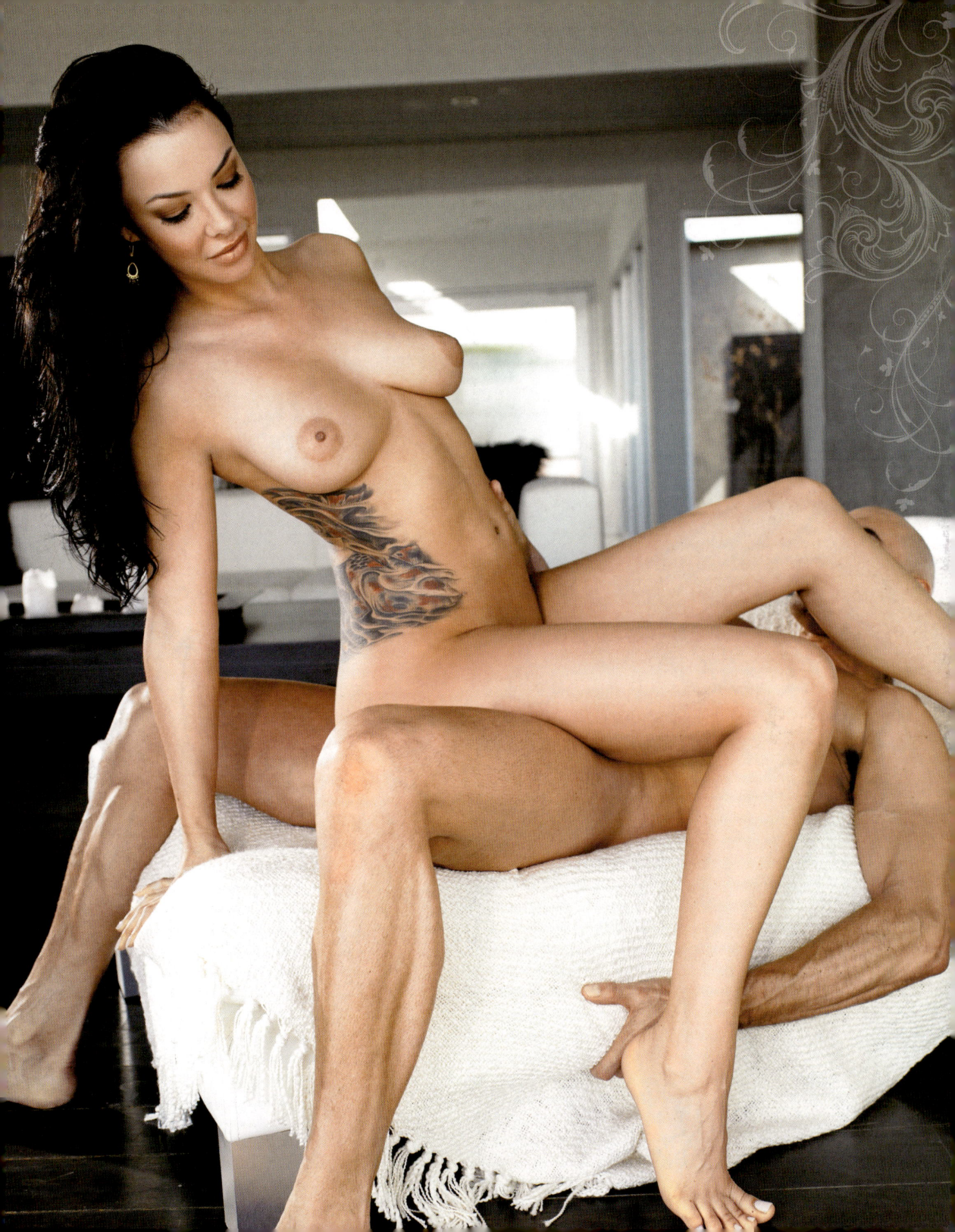

49 | TWINING VINES

{ Entwine Together in the Depths of Pleasure }

IN THIS POSITION, the couple is twined strongly together like vines. It requires a great deal of trust between the partners, because the woman fully releases in a backbend while the man holds her tightly. She needs to have a strong and flexible back, and the man must be confident he can hold her with his upper-body strength. Although the pose may be sustained only briefly, its rewards are great. The backbend opens the woman's upper chakras and rushes energy to her head. The man gets to be deeply embedded inside his woman as he watches her unfurl before him. He must also step into his sacred masculine in order to hold and protect her in her surrendered vulnerability.

① The man is seated on the edge of a chair or bench with his legs apart slightly. The woman sits on his lap facing him, with her legs open wide and her feet flat on either side of him. He wraps his hands around her butt to support her. Here you can kiss passionately, touch each other, and transmit erotic energy to one another by soul gazing. When you are ready, he enters her. You can enjoy intercourse like this for a while, building up the sexual energy.

② When the woman is ready, she begins to straighten out her legs on either side of her lover's body, holding on to his arms for balance. He firmly holds on to her lower back, supporting her as she leans away from him. She uses her abdominal muscles and her hold on his arms to lower herself backward.

The angle of penetration here can feel so good that you may want to stay in this stage for a while before she arches back completely.

③ Eventually the woman leans back completely, wrapping her legs around him, and hangs her head freely (being careful that she has enough room not to hit her head on the floor). To protect the man's back, make sure that he keeps it straight, supporting the woman with the strength of his arms and bending from the hips if necessary, rather than hunching forward or straining his back. From here, he rocks into her gently and she holds on to his thighs for balance as they twine toward orgasmic oneness.

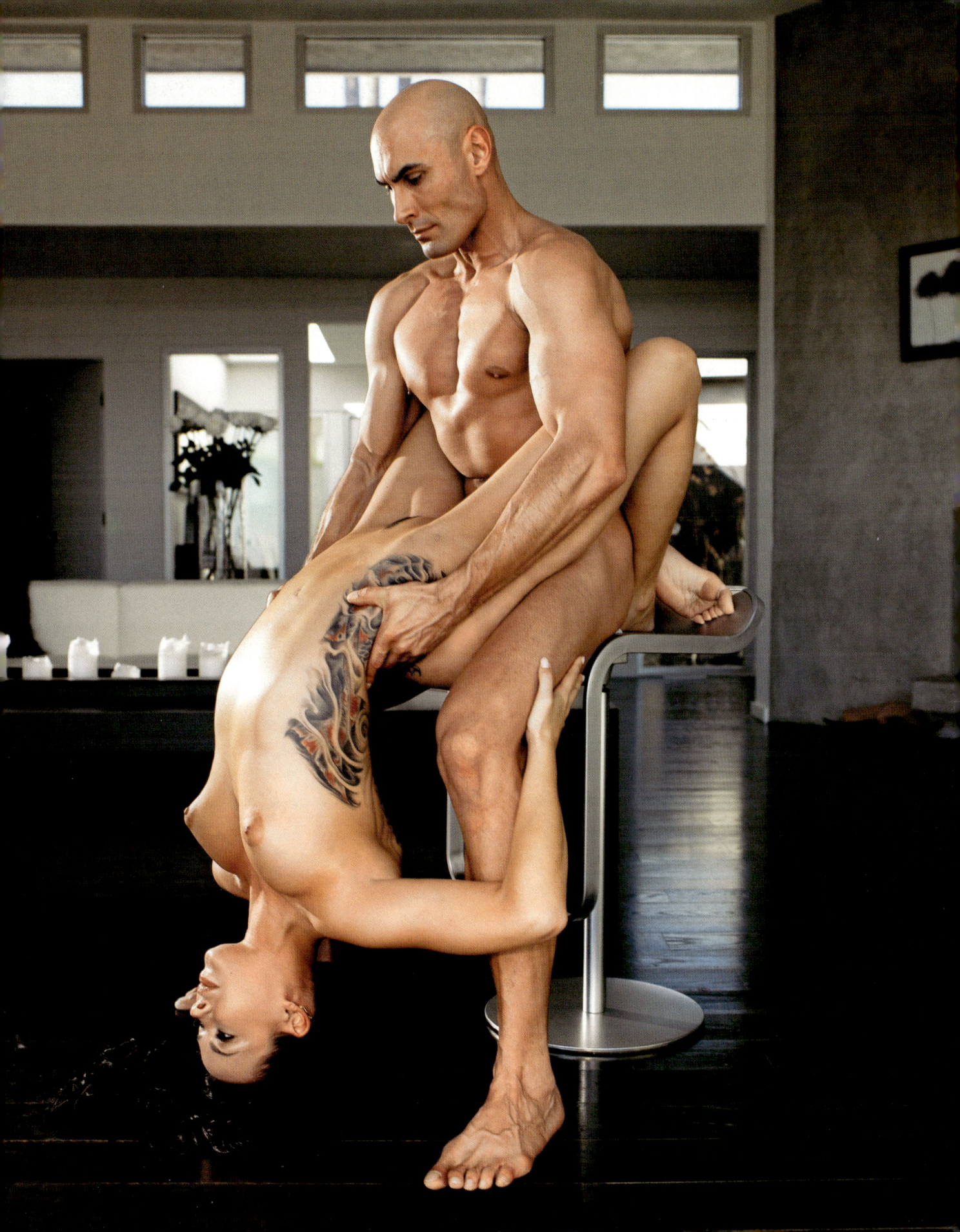

50 | CASCADE

*⊰ A Standing Waterfall
of Intense Sexual Energy ⊱*

IN THIS GRACEFUL SEQUENCE, the woman deeply surrenders in trust to her man as he fills her up with his virility, like water cascading down rocks in a mountain stream. This advanced pose will require strength and flexibility for both partners. The woman should be practiced in and comfortable with backbends and handstands. The man needs complete confidence that he can support them both with his upper-body and leg muscles. Although it may take practice, this posture generates powerful sexually energy by sparking polarity between the masculine and the feminine. Because it requires excellent communication and teamwork, it can be a healing posture for couples coming together after a period of conflict or disconnection.

① Begin by standing and facing one another. The man kneels down on one knee, offering it as a seat to his beloved and opening his arms to welcome her. She sits down on his knee, close to him, wrapping her arms around his neck and partially supporting her weight on the pads of both feet.

② Wrapping his arms around her back tightly, the man uses his leg muscles to slowly come to a standing position. As he does this, the woman wraps her legs around his waist snugly. Bending his knees slightly and engaging his leg muscles to support her weight without straining his back, the man bends forward slightly and lifts her onto his erection. Although movement will be limited, connecting like this can create a strong sexual charge between you. Stay in eye contact and breathe together with a focus on using the breath to complete a circle of energy between you.

③ In the final expression, the man slowly lowers his partner's upper body to the ground and she reaches down into a handstand, supporting herself with her arms as much as possible. She continues to hold on to him with her legs, and he uses his grip around her hips to aid him in filling her with his sacred waters. With all the energy flowing to the crown of her head, the woman may experience orgasm throughout her whole body rather than just in her genitals, whether she enjoys that in the culmination of this posture or experiences it later.

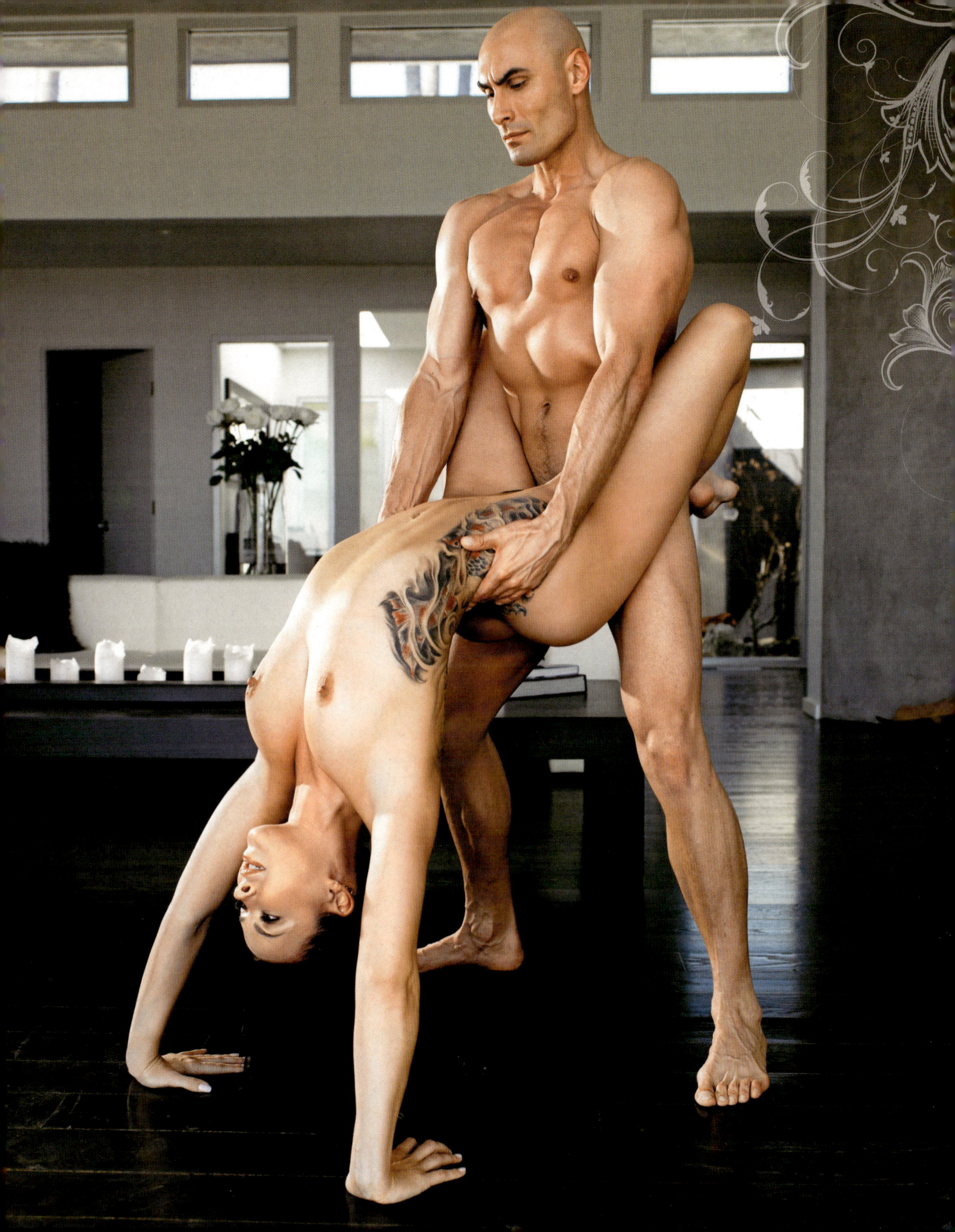

51 ANAL PLAY
52
{ *For Both Him and Her* }

OPEN-MINDED GUY that he was, Vatsyayana mentions anal sex in the Kama Sutra, referring to it as "Lower Congress," although he declines to share any pointers on technique. Long considered taboo, anal play can be extremely erotic (and even orgasmic) for both men and women. In fact, the anus has one of the highest concentrations of nerve endings in the body. Beginning to explore this part of your body can open up a new world of sensual pleasure for you and your partner and may contribute toward reducing stress, promoting healing, and increasing relaxation.

There are many ways to enjoy the anus erotically, and anal sex is just one of them. Many men and women enjoy simply touching the opening or inserting a small toy or finger. These practices benefit both men and women, so take turns giving and receiving. To maximize the pleasure for both of you, it's important to remember the three key points for anal play: communication, relaxation, and lubrication.

If this is something you'd like to explore, either giving, receiving, or both, the first step is *communication*: Talk to your partner. Share your ideas and concerns with one another. Many people think that anal sex has to hurt. That's a dangerous myth and is simply not true. In fact, if it does hurt, tell your partner and stop immediately. Done properly, anal play should feel good. If you're receiving, it's impera-

tive that you communicate openly with your partner about your needs and what you're feeling. If you're giving, check in with your partner frequently and stop immediately if he or she asks you to. Because this is such a sensitive area of the body with so much taboo associated with it, it's normal to feel some uneasiness or discomfort when you first start anal play. But remember that pain shouldn't be part of that.

Relaxation is the second key. There are two rings of muscles in the anus, the external sphincter and the internal sphincter, and they operate independently. The external sphincter can be relaxed at will, but the internal one is controlled by the automatic part of the nervous system. It will tense with fear or stress regardless of how much you might be thinking about relaxing. Breathing deeply, waiting, and being in open communication with your partner will help this muscle relax. It can also be easily "trained" into new behavior. Start by inserting your finger regularly while you shower and the muscle will learn that it's okay to relax. It helps to make an agreement with your partner to just play externally with no penetration for a while to awaken this erogenous zone. In time, you will start to feel more pleasure and be more relaxed.

The third key is *lubrication*. Although the anus produces a small amount of mucus, it does not lubricate like the yoni, so you must always use a

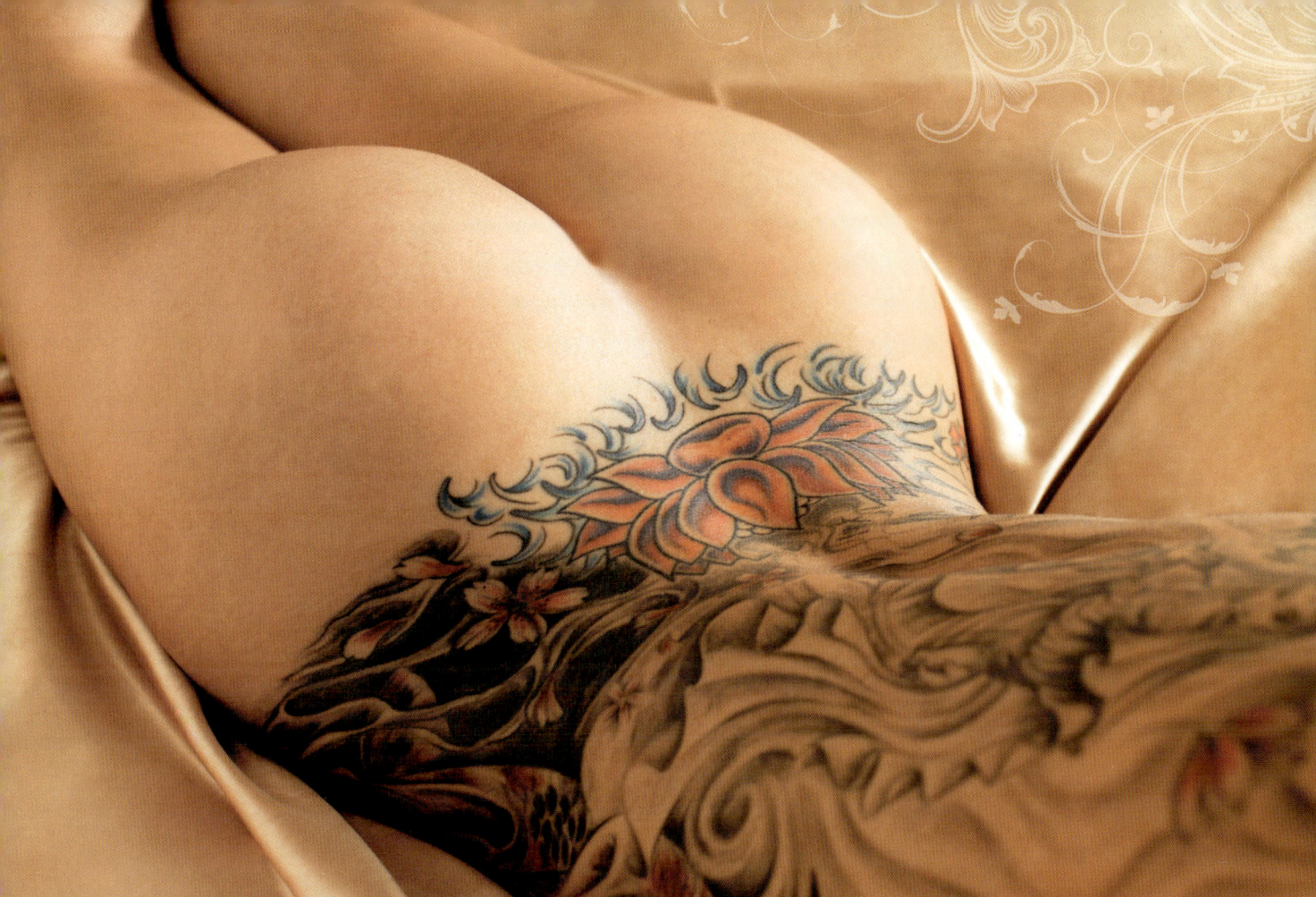

liberal amount of lubrication in anal play and frequently reapply it. Because of the tightness of the fit, the best lubricants are thicker gels.

Part of the taboo with anal play is the "dirty" factor, which turns some people off and turns other people on with its element of the forbidden. It's important to know that with certain precautions, anal play can be completely safe and hygienic. Although the main function of the rectum is as a passageway for feces, it is not normally stored in the rectum except prior to a bowel movement. Make sure you evacuate before play and, of course, wash yourself thoroughly (an enema is not necessary).

A small amount of feces may remain, however, so it's important to *never* switch from anal play to vaginal play without first thoroughly washing the "tool" you're using (whether your finger, a man's vajra, or a toy). One easy way to handle this is to use a condom, latex glove, or a finger cot (a small finger-sized condom available at drug stores), which are easily changed and discarded. Many people also enjoy "rimming," or orally pleasuring the rectum, which can be extremely erotic. If you have an issue with hygiene, you can use a product called a dental dam, an open condom, or even a piece of plastic wrap with some lubricant on the receiver's side to increase sensation and pleasure.

She Receives

Begin by bringing the woman to a heightened state of arousal by stroking and caressing her. For many women, engaging in oral sex or vaginal intercourse prior to anal play can heighten their receptivity and help them feel more open and relaxed. Begin with a well-lubricated finger (or a tongue) and gently apply pressure to her "rosetta" (our Tantric term for anus) without moving. This will help her adjust to the new sensation and relax. The best way for her to relax is not to be afraid about being penetrated too quickly or without her permission. Reassure her that you'll go slowly and stay in communication. When you feel her relaxing, slowly begin moving in a circular motion around the outside of her rosetta, pressing gently without going inside. Ask her if it's okay to go inside, and if she says yes, do that slowly and only go in an inch or so. Remember to stimulate the rest of her body, her breasts and clitoris if possible, to keep her aroused and help her continue to open.

If it feels good to her, you can eventually put a whole finger or two inside her or use a small dildo or a specially shaped anal toy (it will have a flared base to prevent it from going in too deeply and being hard to pull back out). If you are both feeling turned on and ready to try anal sex, be sure to use a lot of lubrication. Even if she desires anal sex and is turned on, remember that the muscles inside the anus can involuntarily contract, which will likely result in pain. If she feels pain upon penetration, be sure to stop all movement and allow her to breathe deeply until the spasm subsides. These can take several minutes. If the man's erection subsides somewhat as well, that can be a benefit. A softer vajra can help her relax and receive you so that when you become erect again she'll be able to feel more pleasure. When she's ready, slowly return to movement or penetration.

All women are different, and even the same woman may have a range of responses and experiences depending on the day. Some women experience strong stimulation of their G-spot through anal penetration and may even reach orgasm. The wall between the anus and the vaginal canal is very thin. For other women, the sensation may not be orgasm inducing, but they're extremely turned on by being taken in such a wanton and taboo way. For others, they crave the intense feeling of being grounded, opened so completely, and filled to overflowing with the juice of their lover.

He Receives

While women routinely have the experience of being penetrated and taking someone or something into their bodies, this is a foreign sensation for most men. Anal play is a powerful way to open new channels of erotic energy in a man and allow him to experience the joys of being penetrated. Enjoying anal play or penetration does not mean that a man is gay! It means he is a healthy, sexually open man who is not afraid to enjoy his body and trusts his partner.

Begin by arousing your man, stroking his vajra and caressing him. If possible, pleasure him orally until you sense he's relaxed and turned on. Check in with him and get permission to play with his rosetta. Start by simply applying gentle pressure without moving using a lubricated finger, a toy, or your tongue. This will help him adjust to your presence there and integrate what he feels. When you sense that he's relaxed, gently move in a circular motion around the outside of his anus. This may be as far as the play goes if you're just beginning. There is a wealth of sensation and pleasure to be had on the outside, so no need to rush anything until you're both very comfortable here.

If he's open and ready, you can insert the tip of a well-lubricated finger and hold it there until his muscles relax. If he's open to more, you can move your finger in a circular motion, and if he's lying on his back, press forward toward the bulb or root of his vajra, which will be pleasurable and stimulating for most men. This is also your access point to his prostate, which is just on the other side of the rectal wall, a few inches in and toward the front of his body. This is known as the male sacred spot, and exploring this part of his body can open up whole new realms of pleasure for him.

For couples who have moved beyond the initial stages of anal play and are ready for more adventure, consider having the woman wear a harness with a dildo attached. Remember the dildo can be any size—the smaller, finger-sized models for anal play are a less threatening way for most men to begin. In this way, a man can bend over a bed or sofa and the woman can penetrate him from behind. This position also enables you to reach around to stroke him manually while he experiences the intense stimulation of having his prostate and the base of his vajra massaged. He just might have the best orgasm of his life.

A warning is due here: it can be highly erotic for a woman to look down and see "her cock" (even if it is plastic and purple). The sensation of thrusting with it (particularly with some strategically placed lubricant between her yoni and the harness) can be quite orgasmic for her. So ladies, remember the three keys of anal play: communication, relaxation, and lubrication. Make sure you stay in good communication with your man and keep in mind that although you might be quite used to being penetrated, it's likely a new experience for him. Go slowly, check in with him often, and don't get carried away (unless, of course, it's mutual.

GLOWING EMBERS

In the afterglow, allow your body to bask in the warmth of your union. Stay connected for as long as possible, nesting, cuddling. Although your body may feel complete for now, your souls remain entwined for quite a while. Continue touching and breathing deeply so that all the energy released by the fire of your passion can integrate into your cells and nourish your deeper union. Don't worry about the cleanup; there's time for that later. Right now, just relax into the love nectar and let it be a blessing from Eros.

And remember the beauty of glowing embers...just the merest breath can cause them to ignite once again.

ACKNOWLEDGMENTS

Thank you to the terrific team at Rockport Publishing and Quiver Books for their invitation to write this book, for making it beautiful, and for providing the world with empowering information about sexuality.

Gratitude to my family and friends for your encouragement and support. I feel so very blessed to have such a loving circle around me. To Mom and Dad, thanks for loving me always, for believing in me, for showing me how to find the Divine in nature, for teaching me to trust feeling good, and for not burdening me with a religious upbringing. To my wise child, Zoe, thanks for filling my heart with your music, for being the brightest star in my sky, and for putting up with all the sex books on the dining room table. To Rick Schlussel, thank you for bringing Zoe into the world with me, for all that we shared, and for beginning the Tantric path with me. To John Hunter, thank you for your editorial support, your giant love, and all the exploration. A special thanks to all the Shakti sisters and coaching clients who've shared their process of awakening and supported my work, particularly my good friends Jennifer Crebbin, Mary Beauchamp, and Diane Giuliani.

To Karin Tobiason for the companionship of your writer's soul, your friendship, and intuitive insights. To Felicia Eth for your guidance. To Helen Neff and Grass Valley Bikram Yoga for the discipline, balance, and flow of the practice—it has contributed immeasurably to my life and this book. To Kali Ma Troma Rinpoche, for being such an inspiration and for bringing the MahaSiddha Dharma to us with such humor, compassion, fierceness, and love.